HEALTHY SMOOTHIE RECIPES

Super Food Smoothies for Weight Loss, Detox, and Improved Health

(Gain Energy, Lose Weight, Detox and Feel Stronger)

Michael Howe

Published by Alex Howard

© Michael Howe

All Rights Reserved

Healthy Smoothie Recipes: Super Food Smoothies for Weight Loss, Detox, and Improved Health (Gain Energy, Lose Weight, Detox and Feel Stronger)

ISBN 978-1-990169-81-6

Legal & Disclaimer

The information contained in this book is not designed to replace or take the place of any form of medicine or professional medical advice. The information in this book has been provided for educational and entertainment purposes only.

Table of contents

Part 1

Introduction

The keto diet is well known for its great ability to turn the body into a fat burning machine.

For those looking to lose weight and improve their overall health, the Ketogenic diet is a great tool to turn to. As with any diet or eating plan though, it is essential to be a little organised, so you are able to stick to eating the correct foods and to stay focused. Making sure you are still consuming a wealth of vitamins and minerals and avoiding carbohydrates can be a challenge, which is where we can help.

Our collection of delicious smoothies & juices have been designed to complement your existing Keto diet. Most are green but we've sneaked in a few mixed smoothies too to add some variety. Some of our smoothies can be used as a meal replacement, if your goal is weight loss and therefore each is calorie counted, however we suggest our smoothies are best used as part of your overall Keto eating plan.

Devised to detox your body we suggest you consume 2-3 smoothies from the detox and energising chapters of this book for 10 consecutive days as part of your balanced daily Keto diet. This will help rid your body of unwanted and harmful toxins and leave you feeling energised and cleansed whilst setting you on a path to sustained weight loss. The final chapter 'Full Keto' will keep you inspired long term. You should introduce smoothies from this chapter after your initial 10 day detox period.

But what is Keto?
There are numerous types of Keto eating plans out there, but Ketogenic Green Smoothies follows basic, standard principles; working on the belief that the body benefits from eating easy to digest and unprocessed foods is important, plus consuming minimal carbohydrate and high levels of animal-based proteins, natural plant fats, vegetables, nuts and seeds is the core of a Keto diet.

Essentially this method is aimed to programme the body to use its unwanted stores of fat, instead of burning the sugary carbohydrates that are more usually consumed. By restricting these carbohydrates, you begin to re-programme your body to use the fat stores, instead of the glycogen stores in the muscles – this process is known as ketosis.

Once you have hit 'full' Ketosis and your body is in this high gear, you will find your metabolism is increased and the quality of the Keto food you consume will provide you with lots of energy and more mental alertness. Afternoon "slumps" are less likely to be experienced due to the fact you are eating adequate nutrition. Ordinarily reducing calories to achieve weight loss can result in low moods and agitation however this too can be avoided when eating a Keto diet as you will be reducing carbohydrates but not reducing calories and nutrition!

How Do You Know You're in Full Ketosis?
When your body is functioning at this level it is breaking down Ketones (fats and fatty acids) for energy, rather than the glucose from carbohydrates. As a result you should experience the following:

* Excess weight loss
* Loss of appetite
* Increased focus and energy
* Less energy dips
* Increased urination

The Potential Benefits?
The Ketogenic Diet brings many benefits to your health and long term, it can really help with chronic health issues.

* Reduction in weight
* Lowered insulin levels and reduced risk of developing Type II Diabetes
* Clearer skin
* Better control of epilepsy
* Increased levels of good cholesterol
* Lower blood pressure
* Reduced risk of developing brain disease.

What to Eat?

Protein such as beef, lamb, pork, chicken, venison, fish, seafood & tofu. Try to use grass fed, organic and sustainably sourced where possible.

Eggs: Organic

Dairy Products: full fat and organic, real butter, cream and cheeses. Always avoid low fat, sugary varieties.

Vegetables: asparagus, spinach, all types of cabbage, mushrooms, peppers, tomatoes, cucumber, olives, courgette, aubergine, etc.

Nuts and Seeds: almonds, macadamia, brazil nuts, hazelnuts, walnuts, pumpkin seeds, chia seeds, sesame seeds, sunflower seeds, etc.

Fruits: raspberries, blueberries, strawberries and blackberries (only in moderation though and exclude if you are on a weight loss goal).

Natural Fats: avocado oil, sesame oil, olive oil and coconut oil.

Drinks: coconut water, tea and coffee, with cream.

Foods to avoid include: starchy root vegetables; processed food; sugary food; energy drinks; grains & beans.

Ketogenic Green Smoothies make life easy by helping keep you inspired with a broad spectrum of vital plant compounds and animal-based proteins to complement your overall keto eating plan.

Notes On Blenders

There are many high-speed blenders out there on the market of various designs. Many have an upside-down cup and described as a "bullet" and some come with extra cups and drinks tops. They take up minimal space in the cupboard or on a work surface, for quick access. This makes creating smoothies and healthy drinks so easy to work into a busy schedule.

Many vegetable smoothies and juices taste even better iced cold. These blender "bullets" are great at smashing through ice cubes to add to your drink, to create some lovely crushed ice concoctions.
It's worth investing in a good quality appliance. When you use a kitchen appliance daily, it's usually worth every penny spent! However, all of these recipes can still be made in a food processor of most designs, so there is no need to purchase expensive gadgets when getting started. Use the smallest bowl ones and soak the nuts or seeds overnight if possible, to help make processing the ingredients a little less work.

Tips On Blending
To make the most of your blending, follow these tips:
* Always use the freshest ingredients possible.
* Chop ingredients, especially harder produce, into small pieces to ensure
smoother blending.
* Wash vegetables and fruit really well before use.

* Once a smoothie or drink has been processed, it will begin to lose its nutritional value, so it is best to consume as soon as possible after being made.

* If you want to prepare ahead, add everything to the blender cup and store in the fridge until the last minute and then blend just before needed.

* You can use a variety of frozen fruits and vegetables for these recipes. It will make the drinks icy cold and sometimes quite "slushie" which is great for a hot day or for after a hard work out!

* You can freeze avocados to be used for smoothies (their texture after freezing is not suitable for slicing on to a dish). You can remove the stone, peel and then mash half an avocado with a little lemon juice. Store these individually in little freezer bags so you can remove as and when you need for single portions.

* Adding ½ tsp of coconut oil to smoothies and drinks can be a welcome addition if you wish to increase the fat content a little in your Keto diet. When stored at a reasonably warm room temperature, the oil will almost be a liquid so easy to reach for and spoon out.

* If you find you can't get all of the ingredients into your blender in one go, add some of them and then blend to make room. Add the rest and continue.

* Make sure the blender is unplugged before disassembling or cleaning.

Set aside the power base and blade holders as these should not be used in a dishwasher.

*Use hot soapy water to clean the blades but do not immerse in boiling water as this can warp the plastic.

* Use a damp cloth to clean the power base.
* All cups and lids can be placed in a dishwasher.
* For stubborn marks inside the cup, fill the cup 2/3 full of warm soapy water and screw on the milling blade. Attached to the power base and run for 20-30 seconds.
* During cleaning or use do not put your hands or any utensils near the moving blade. Always ensure the blender/food processor is unplugged when assembling/disassembling or cleaning.

The type of blender you have will dictate which seeds and skins should be removed from fruit and vegetables. However the following seeds and pits should always be removed before blending as they may contain chemicals which can release cyanide into the body when ingested so do not use any of the following in your smoothies:

* **Apple Seeds**
* **Cherry Pits**
* **Peach pits**
* **Apricot Pits**
* **Plum Pits**

The different drinks and smoothies in Ketogenic Green Smoothies are split into three categories: Detox, Energising and Full Keto which give you a choice of recipes depending on your mood or requirements.

Detox

This section gives you a number of drink recipes using water or coconut water as a base. Coconut water is a natural, hydrating drink which provides calcium, phosphorus, magnesium, sodium and potassium. It is the drink of choice for many athletes and is a great choice to blend with foods to produce nutritious drinks.

Allowing the body to rest from working hard to remove toxins from our body, is essential for our health. This can be done by eliminating as many toxic foods from your diet as possible and also by consuming the vegetables and herbs that will assist your body with the detoxification process. Cleansing and hydrating drinks with natural ingredients from many different sources is a great addition to a Keto diet.

Energising
This section has a wealth of recipes to inspire you to keep to your dietary objectives. When faced with inadequate nutrition, it is easy to reach for foods that are restricted just because it is easy. These energising drinks will provide you with energy and proteins, needed for repair and growth, so you remain positive and full of vitality.

Many of these drinks use unsweetened almond milk, coconut milk, nuts, seeds and nut butters as a base and provide the essential good fats needed on a Keto diet. They will keep you feeling fuller for longer and some of these could be used as meal replacements if you are trying to lose weight. Give some of these flavour combinations a go, as you may be surprised.

Full Keto

These drinks are aimed towards those who have settled into a great Keto eating plan and have embraced the changes. Using ingredients that are typically high in animal proteins and fats and some ingredients that should only be eaten in moderation, these drinks provide some well-loved flavours. Life is short and whatever eating plan you follow, everyone loves a treat from time to time (note: if you are on a weight loss programme, you may only want to dip into these recipes occasionally).

Many of these drinks use single cream, but this can be substituted with whipping cream or even cream cheese and sour cream. Try to aim for dairy creams that are 40% fat and higher for the best results.

Ketogenic Green Smoothies is inspiration and motivation to keep adequately hydrated and nourished whilst eating a Keto diet. Yes, there are a number of foods that need to be avoided, but you can celebrate and enjoy the foods you CAN eat. Try out some of these great flavour combinations knowing they have been designed to taste great and to give your wellbeing a well-deserved boost.

About CookNation
CookNation is the leading publisher of innovative and practical recipe books for the modern, health conscious cook.

CookNation titles bring together delicious, easy and practical recipes with their unique no-nonsense approach - making cooking for diets and healthy eating fast, simple and fun. With a range of #1 best-selling titles - from the innovative 'Skinny' calorie-counted series, to the 5:2 Diet Recipes collection - CookNation recipe books prove that 'Diet' can still mean 'Delicious'!

Detox Green Smoothies

Detox Kale & Celery

Serves 1
190 calories

Ingredients
225g/8oz kale
1 stalk off celery
250ml/8½floz coconut water
Avocado
1 tbsp fresh flat leaf parsley
Water

Method
Rinse the kale and remove any thick stalks.

Rinse the celery well.
Add all of the ingredients into a high speed blender.
Add a little water if needed to make up to the level that will fill your smoothie glass.
Blend the ingredients together until really smooth. Enjoy immediately.

Chef's Note
Celery is believed to cleanse the blood.

Warm Spice Cleanse

Serves 1
155 calories

Ingredients
75g/3oz kale
250ml/8½floz coconut water
150g/5oz yellow or orange bell pepper
Pinch of cumin
½ tbsp fresh grated ginger
½ tsp turmeric (fresh or ground)
Water

Method
Rinse the kale and remove any thick stalks
Rinse the bell pepper and remove any seeds. Roughly chop.
Add all the ingredients to a high-speed blender and top up with enough water if needed, to make up to the level to fill your smoothie glass.

Process the ingredients until really smooth. Enjoy immediately.

Chef's Note
Peppers are packed with anti-oxidants.

Gardener's Cleanse

Serves 1
259 calories

Ingredients
50g/2oz baby beetroot leaves
50g/2oz baby spinach leaves
250ml/8½floz coconut water
1 tbsp fresh flat leaf parsley
75g/3oz courgette
50g/2oz whole almonds
Water

Method
Rinse the baby leaves well and drain.
Rinse the courgette and roughly chop. Leave the skin and seeds intact.
Add everything to a high-speed blender.
Top with a little water if need be, so the level will fill your smoothie glass.
Blend the ingredients really well until smooth. Enjoy immediately.

Chef's Note

Parsley is associated with helping the kidneys and liver to detox.

Fresh Green Cleanse

Serves 1
230 calories

Ingredients
2 celery stalks
300g/11oz cucumber
125g/4oz kale
225g/8oz spinach
1 tbsp fresh coriander
1 lemon
1 lime
Water

Method
Wash the celery, spinach, cucumber, coriander and drain.
Cut any thick green stalks off the kale and rinse well.
Peel and de-seed the lemon and lime.
Add all of the ingredients to a high-speed blender and add enough water to a level that will fill your smoothie glass.
Process the ingredients until smooth. Enjoy immediately.

Chef's Note

Coriander is known to support liver function and is a great detox ingredient.

Super Green Slush

Serves 1
116 calories

Ingredients
125g/4oz cucumber
50g/2oz baby spinach leaves
1 tbsp fresh mint leaves
250ml/8½floz coconut water
1 tbsp lemon juice
2 handfuls of ice

Method
Rinse the spinach and drain well.
Rinse the cucumber and roughly chop but leave the skin and seeds intact.
Rinse the mint leaves.
Add all of the ingredients into a high-speed blender.
Process the ingredients until quite smooth but still icy and fresh.
Enjoy immediately

Chef's Note
Mint is a great in a detox drink, it's fresh tasting and full of soothing properties.

Detox Italian

Serves 1
123 calories

Ingredients
100g/3½oz aubergine
4 black olives
250ml/8 ½floz coconut water
1 tsp rosemary leaves
1 small garlic clove
Water

Method
Rinse and roughly chop the aubergine
Crush the garlic clove.
Add all of the ingredients into a high-speed blender and add enough water to a level that will fill your smoothie glass.
Process the ingredients until smooth. This may take a little longer to ensure the rosemary is broken down. Enjoy immediately.

Chef's Note
Rosemary is known to both help the liver detox and to improve brain function.

Yellow Ginger Cleanse

Serves 1
128 calories

Ingredients
2cm/1 inch fresh root ginger
150g/5oz kale
125g/4oz broccoli
250ml/8½floz coconut water
½ tsp turmeric
Water

Method
Prepare the ginger and grate into the cup of a high speed blender.
Rinse the broccoli and cut into small pieces.
Add all of the ingredients into the blender and top up with enough water to a level that will fill your smoothie glass.
Blend until the ingredients are really smooth.
Enjoy immediately.

Chef's Note
The turmeric adds a lovely yellow hue to this drink and has anti-inflammatory benefits.

Bamboo Hydrator

Serves 1
120 calories

Ingredients
175g/6oz bamboo shoots
200g/7 oz bok choi

125g/4oz cucumber
250ml/8½floz coconut water
3-4 fennel seeds
Water

Method
Drain and rinse the bamboo shoots (if using canned)
Rinse the bok choi and roughly chop.
Rinse the cucumber and roughly chop, leaving the skin and seeds intact,
Add all the ingredients into a high-speed blender and top up with enough water to reach a level that will fill your smoothie glass.
Process the ingredients until really smooth. Enjoy immediately.

Chef's Note
Bamboo shoots are a great source of fibre that is sometimes hard to find on a keto diet.

Vitamin C Booster

Serves 1
193 calories

Ingredients
175g/6oz red bell pepper
125g/4 oz kale
200ml/7floz coconut water
1 tsp grated ginger root
½ tsp turmeric

Water

Method
Rinse the bell pepper and roughly chop, removing the seeds.
Rinse the kale and remove any thick stems.
Prepare the ginger root and grate in to a blender.
Add all of the other ingredients in to the blender and top up with enough water so the level will fill you glass.
Process the ingredients until really smooth. Enjoy immediately.

Chef's Note
Red bell peppers and kale together provide wonderful sources of vitamin C, essential to see you through cold season.

Baby Leaf Hydrator
Serves 1
94 calories

Ingredients
75g/3oz baby beetroot leaves
75g/3oz baby spinach leaves
250ml/8½floz coconut water
1 tbsp flat leaf parsley leaves
3-4 whole almonds
Water

Method

Rinse the baby leaves and parsley, drain well.,
Roughly chop the almonds to help the processing a little.
Add all of the ingredients into a high-speed blender and top with enough water to bring to a level to fill your glass.
Process the ingredients until really smooth. Enjoy immediately.

Chef's Note
The baby leaves used in this drink will help improve calcium levels.

Mint And Watercress Detox

Serves 1
90 calories

Ingredients
150g/5oz watercress leaves
1 tbsp mint leaves
250ml/8½floz coconut water
75g/3oz asparagus spears
Water

Method
Rinse the watercress and mint well, Drain.
Clean the asparagus and roughly chop, removing any really fibrous stem.

Place the ingredients into a high-speed blender and top up with enough water to enable you to fill your glass.
Blend the ingredients until really smooth.
Enjoy immediately.

Chef's Note
Watercress provides a great source of vitamin C and can help fight illness.

The Green Machine
Serves 1
136 calories

Ingredients
125g/4oz cucumber
1 celery stalk
150g/5oz kale
250ml/8½floz coconut water
1 tbsp lemon juice
1 tbsp lime juice
1 tbsp coriander leaves
Water

Method
Rinse the cucumber and roughly chop, leaving the seeds and skin intact.
Rinse the kale and remove any thick stems.
Rinse and drain the coriander leaves.

Add all of the ingredients into a high-speed blender and top up with enough water to fill the glass you are using,
Blend the ingredients really well and until smooth. Enjoy immediately.

Chef's Note
The added coriander can also help ease indigestion and bloating.

Broccoli Salad Detox

Serves 1
145 calories

Ingredients
150g/5oz broccoli
150g/5oz romaine lettuce leaves
75g/3oz baby spinach leaves
1 tbsp oregano
250ml/8½floz coconut water
Water

Method
Rinse and roughly chop the broccoli florets.
Rinse and drain the romaine, spinach and oregano leaves
Add all of the ingredients into a high-speed blender and top up with enough extra water to fill a smoothie glass.

Process the ingredients until well blended. Enjoy immediately.

Chef's Note
Broccoli is a vegetable that really benefits the blood. It provides Vitamin K, which improves blood clotting,

Red Radish Detox
Serves 1
108 calories

Ingredients
200g/7oz red radishes
150g/5oz white cabbage
1 tbsp thyme leaves
250ml/8½floz coconut water
Water

Method
Rinse the radishes and remove the green stalks on each.
Rinse and core the cabbage and roughly chop.
Rinse and drain the thyme.
Add everything to a high-speed blender and add enough water to fill the glass you are using.
Process all of the ingredients until smooth.
Enjoy immediately.

Chef's Note
Vitamin E is an essential nutrient to balance hormones.

Garlic Cleanser

Serves 1
111 calories

Ingredients
200g/7oz cauliflower
1 garlic clove
50g courgette
1 tsp lemon juice
250ml/8½floz coconut water
1 tbsp parsley
Water

Method
Rinse the cauliflower well and roughly chop.
Rinse the courgette and roughly chop, leaving the skin and seeds intact.
Wash the parsley leaves and drain well.
Add all of the ingredients into a high speed blender and top up with water to make enough liquid to fill your glass.
Blend the ingredients together until smooth. Enjoy immediately.

Chef's Note
Garlic is known for its great anti-oxidant abilities, maybe chew some mint leaves after though!

Alfalfa Herbal Detox

Serves 1
89 calories

Ingredients
75g/3oz alfalfa sprouts
2 stalks of celery
1 tsp sage leaves
1 tsp thyme
1 tbsp lemon juice
250ml/8½floz coconut water
Water

Method
Rinse the alfalfa really well and drain.
Rinse the celery stalks and roughly chop.
Rinse the herbs and drain.
Add everything to a high-speed blender and top up with water so there is enough liquid to fill your glass.
Blend until really smooth. Enjoy immediately.

Chef's Note
It is thought that alfalfa sprouts have great anti-ageing and anti-oxidant benefits.

Asparagus Refresher

Serves 1
110 calories

Ingredients
150g/5oz asparagus
125g/4oz cucumber
250ml/8½floz coconut water
1 lemon
1 tbsp flat leaf parsley leaves
Ice cubes

Method
Wash and roughly chop the asparagus, removing any fibrous stems at the end.
Wash and roughly chop the cucumber, leaving skin and seeds intact.
Wash and peel the lemon.
Wash and drain the parsley.
Add all of the ingredients into a high-speed blender.
When smooth, add handfuls of ice and process again, to create a hydrating, slushie drink.

Chef's Note
Asparagus can help detoxify the liver and kidneys and has a generally cleansing effect on your body's other systems.

Herbal Detox Juice

Serves 1
142 calories

Ingredients

50g/2oz kale
150g/5oz courgette
1 stalk of celery
1 tbsp flat leaf parsley
1 tbsp oregano leaves
5 black olives, pitted
200ml/7floz coconut water
1 tbsp lemon juice
Water

Method
Rinse the kale and celery.
Cut the thick stems from the kale and roughly chop.
Rinse and roughly chop the courgette, leaving the skin and seeds intact.
Rinse the parsley and oregano, drain.
Add all of the ingredients into a high-speed blender and add a little water if need be.
Process until the ingredients are smooth. Enjoy immediately.

Chef's Note
Oregano and parsley are both diuretics that help flush toxins from your body.

Tomato Detox

Serves 1
126 calories

Ingredients

150g plum tomatoes
250ml/8½ coconut water
100g/3½oz aubergine
1 garlic clove
1 tbsp basil leaves
Water and ice

Method
Rinse the tomatoes and roughly chop.
Rinse the aubergine and roughly chop.
Crush the garlic clove and add it to a high-speed blender.
Rinse the basil and drain.
Add all of the ingredients to the blender and top up with water if need be, so the level fills the glass you are using.
Blend the ingredients until smooth. This smoothie is particularly nice with lots of crushed ice. Enjoy immediately.

Chef's Note
Tomatoes are a great source of lycopene, a useful anti-oxidant which aids detox.

Sauerkraut & Dill Cleanse
Serves 1
143 calories

Ingredients
60g/2½oz sauerkraut
100g/3½oz cauliflower
250ml/8½floz coconut water
1 lemon
1 tbsp fresh dill
water

Method
Drain the sauerkraut well.
Rinse the cauliflower and roughly chop in to small florets.
Wash the dill and drain,
Peel and roughly chop the lemon.
Add all of the ingredients into a high-speed blender, topping up with water if necessary so you can fill your glass.
Process the ingredients until smooth. Enjoy immediately,

Chef's Note
Sauerkraut is full of beta-carotene which works as a great anti-oxidant. It is known to improve gut bacteria and helpful during a detox.

Sprout Top Smoothie
Serves 1
185 calories

Ingredients

125g/4 Brussels sprout tops
125g/4oz cauliflower
125g/4oz cucumber
1 tbsp coriander leaves
250ml/8½floz coconut water
1 tbsp lemon juice
Water

Method
Rinse the Brussels sprout tops and drain. Roughly chop.
Wash and roughly chop the cauliflower.
Rinse the cucumber and roughly chop, leaving the skin and seeds intact.
Add all of the ingredients to a high-speed blender and add a little more water, to reach the level that will fill your glass.
Blend until all of the ingredients are smooth. Enjoy immediately,

Chef's Note
Brussels sprout tops aren't widely used but are a cheap way to pack your diet with Vitamin C, perfect for a detox programme.

Lemon Verbena & Cucumber Cleanser
Serves 1
118 calories

Ingredients

3 tbsp lemon verbena leaves
150g/5oz cucumber
2 stalks of celery
250ml/8½floz coconut water
1 tsp mint leaves
Water and ice

Method

Rinse and drain the lemon verbena and mint leaves.
Wash and roughly chop the cucumber, leaving the skin and seeds intact.
Wash and roughly chop the celery leaves.
Place all of the ingredients into a high-speed blender and add a little more water if need be, to make up to the level of your glass.
Process all of the ingredients until smooth. Add a large handful of ice if desired. Enjoy immediately.

Chef's Note

Lemon verbena can offer protection against oxidative stress and has been studied at length to suggest it has great anti-oxidant properties.

Mediterranean Detox

Serves 1
167 calories

Ingredients

150g yellow/orange bell pepper

250ml/8½floz coconut water
75g/3oz rocket leaves
100g/3½oz plum tomatoes
1 tsp rosemary leaves
Ice cubes

Method
Wash and de-seed the pepper. Roughly chop.
Wash the rocket and rosemary leaves and drain well.
Wash the tomatoes and roughly chop.
Add all of the ingredients into a high-speed blender and top up with water if need be, to fill the glass you are using,
Blend until all of the ingredients are smooth. Enjoy immediately.

Chef's Note
The essential carotenoids found in peppers are essential for protection against free radicals.

Green Leaf Cleanser

Serves 1
204 calories

Ingredients
125g/4oz rocket leaves
50g/2oz spinach leaves
50g/2oz butterhead lettuce
250ml/8½floz coconut water
1 tsp spirulina

1 tbsp pumpkin seeds
Water

Method
Rinse the rocket, spinach and butterhead and drain well.
Add all the ingredients to a high-speed blender and add a little more water if needed, to make up to fill the glass you are using.
Blend until really smooth. Enjoy immediately.

Chef's Note
Spirulina is a form of blue-green algae with powerful healing and cleansing properties.

Chia, Lime & Mint Detox
Serves 1
185 calories

Ingredients
100g/3½oz cucumber
250ml/8½floz coconut water
1 lime
3 tbsp mint leaves
1 tbsp chia seeds
Water

Method
Wash the cucumber and roughly chop, leaving the skin and seeds intact.

Peel the lime and roughly chop.

Wash and drain the mint leaves.

Add all of the ingredients into a high-speed blender, adding a little more water if necessary to make up to the level to fill the glass you are using.

Process the ingredients until smooth. You can enjoy this drink 1-2 hours after making it as the soaking chia seeds will create a thicker texture, if you prefer.

Chef's Note

Chia seeds contain high amounts of both soluble and insoluble fibre, and help to clean out the digestive tract.

Cauliflower Cleanser

Serves 1

162 calories

Ingredients

150g/5oz cauliflower

2 stalks of celery

125g/4oz white cabbage

250ml/8½floz coconut water

2 tbsp chives

Water

Method

Wash the cauliflower and cut in to small florets.

Wash and roughly chop the celery and cabbage.

Wash the chives and drain well.
Place all of the ingredients in to a high-speed blender and add a little more water if needed, to make up to the level needed to fill the glass you are using.
Process the ingredients until smooth, Enjoy immediately.

Chef's Note
The glucosinolates in cauliflower activate the detoxification enzymes in our bodies.

Watercress & Lemon Zinger
Serves 1
194 calories

Ingredients
250ml/8½floz coconut water
150g/5oz watercress
1 lemon
125g/4oz spinach
Water

Method
Rinse the watercress and spinach well and drain.
Add all the ingredients to a high-speed blender and add a little more water if need be, to make up to the level of the glass you are using.
Blend the ingredients until really smooth. Enjoy immediately.

Chef's Note

High in antioxidants, nutrients and vitamin C, watercress is a great detox ingredient.

Asian Green Detox

Serves 1
135 calories

Ingredients

100g/3½oz mangetout
100g/3½oz bok choi
250ml/8½floz coconut water
50g/2oz bamboo shoots
1 pinch of Chinese 5 spice
1 tsp grated fresh ginger

Method

Rinse and drain the mangetout and roughly chop.
Wash the bok choi and drain and split the leaves.
Rinse the bamboo shoots well.
Add all of the ingredients into a high-speed blender, adding a little water to make up to the level that will fill the glass you are using.
Blend the ingredients until smooth. Enjoy immediately.

Chef's Note

Bok choi is a source of quercetin, which is a powerful phytonutrient for removing free radicals from the body.

Country Garden Cleanse

Serves 1
251 calories

Ingredients
150g/5oz Brussels sprout tops
50g/2oz spinach leaves
125g/4oz courgette
1 tsp sage leaves
1 tsp wheatgrass
Water

Method
Rinse the Brussels sprout tops and spinach leaves. Roughly chop.
Wash and roughly chop the courgette, leaving the skin and seeds intact.
Wash the sage leaves and drain well.
Add all of the ingredients into a high-speed blender, adding a bit more water to make up the level to fill your glass.
Blend until smooth. Enjoy immediately.

Chef's Note
Wheatgrass is a great detox ingredient and will boost your diet with chlorophyll, to help remove toxins.

Cleansing Goji

Serves 1

172 calories

Ingredients
1 tbsp dried goji berries
1 tsp ginger root, grated
125g/4oz spinach leaves
250ml/8½floz green tea, cooled
Water
Ice

Method
Soak the goji berries in a little water for around 15 minutes.
Rinse and drain the spinach leaves.
Place all of the ingredients into a high-speed blender and top up with a little water if you want a longer drink.
Process the ingredients until smooth.
Serve with plenty of ice.

Chef's Note
Goji berries are a wonderful superfood - they're packed with antioxidants, vitamins, minerals and fibre.

Kale & Fennel Boost

Serves 1
190 calories

Ingredients
140g/4½oz kale

250ml/8½floz coconut water
2 stalks of celery
125g/4oz of cucumber
4-5 fennel seeds
1 tsp flat leaf parsley
1 tbsp lemon juice
Water

Method
Rinse the kale well and remove any thick stalks.
Rinse the celery and roughly chop.
Clean and roughly chop the cucumber, keeping the seeds and skin intact.
Rinse the parsley and crush the fennel seeds a bit.
Add all of the ingredients into a high-speed blender, topping up with water to fill the glass you are using.
Blend until really smooth. Enjoy immediately.

Chef's Note
Kale is believed to help prevent cardiovascular disease, several types of cancer, asthma, rheumatoid arthritis, and premature ageing of the skin.

Rocket Booster
Serves 1
100 calories

Ingredients
250ml/8½floz coconut water
200g/7oz rocket leaves

2 tbsp lime juice
150g/5oz courgette
½ tsp oregano leaves
water

Method
Rinse and drain the rocket the leaves.
Rinse the courgette and roughly chop, leaving the skin and seeds intact.
Wash the oregano leaves and drain.
Add all of the ingredients into a high-speed blender, topping up with water if necessary.
Blend the ingredients well until smooth. Enjoy immediately.

Chef's Note
Rocket leaves contain anti-oxidants that cleanse toxins and they will give you a boost of vitamin C.

Energising Green Smoothies

Mighty Nut Aubergine

Serves 1
246 calories

Ingredients
125g/4oz aubergine
1 tbsp walnuts

125g/4oz spinach
2 tbsp full fat Greek yogurt
100ml/3½floz coconut water
Water

Method
Wash the spinach and aubergine,
Roughly chop the aubergine and walnuts.
Add the ingredients into a high-speed blender and top up with water so the level will fill the glass you are using.
Blend the ingredients until really smooth. Enjoy immediately.

Chef's Note
Walnuts are a great source of omega-3, the good fat that will boost energy.

Spinach Power
Serves 1
290 calories

Ingredients
150g/5oz spinach leaves
50g/2oz mangetout
½ avocado
4 tbsp low fat Greek yogurt
1 tbsp mint leaves
100ml/3½floz coconut water
Water

2 tsp honey

Method
Rinse the spinach leaves, mint and mangetout.
Peel and remove the stone from the avocado.
Add all of the ingredients into a high-speed blender and add water if needed, so to fill the glass you will be using.
Blend the ingredients until really smooth. Enjoy immediately.

Chef's Note
Spinach is a good source of iron that will boost your red blood cells and the oxygen levels in your blood.

Energy Seed Smoothie

Serves 1
287 calories

Ingredients
175ml/6floz almond milk
1 tbsp pumpkin seeds
1 tbsp chia seeds
75g/3oz broccoli
75g/3oz courgette
2 tbsp full fat Greek yogurt
Water

Method
Rinse the broccoli and roughly chop.

Rinse the courgette and roughly chop, leaving the skin and seeds intact.
Add all the ingredients into a high-speed blender and top up with water if necessary, so it will fill the glass you are using.
Process the ingredients until really smooth. Enjoy immediately.

Chef's Note
Seeds are an excellent way to get some good fats and energy into a keto diet. Whilst relatively low in carbohydrates, they still pack a punch!

Flax Power Smoothie

Serves 1
231 calories

Ingredients
75g/3oz radishes
½ avocado
2 tbsp flat leaf parsley
2 tbsp flaxseed
250ml/8½floz unsweetened almond milk
Water

Method
Wash the radishes and remove the green ends.
Remove the stone and peel the avocado.
Wash and drain the parsley leaves.

Put all of the ingredients into a high-speed blender and add a little water if needed, so the level will fill the glass you are using.
Process the ingredients until smooth. Enjoy immediately.

Chef's Note
Flaxseeds are a superfood well known for their nutrients and health benefits. They are a great protein to add to a
Keto diet to give you a boost in energy.

Berry Hemp Blend
Serves 1
346 calories

Ingredients
½ avocado
125g/4oz raspberries
120ml/4floz unsweetened almond milk
2 tbsp full fat Greek Yoghurt
1 tbsp hemp seeds
Water

Method
Rinse the raspberries.
Remove the peel and stone from the avocado.
Place all of the ingredients into a high-speed blender and add a little water if need be, so to fill the glass you are using.

Process the ingredients until smooth. Enjoy immediately.

Chef's Note
Berries should be used in moderation when following a Keto plan, but they can offer a welcome sweetness from time to time and they balance the flavours of the hemp seed here well,

Cacao Superfood Smoothie
Serves 1
305 calories

Ingredients
250ml/8½floz coconut water
50g/2oz avocado
1 tbsp chia seeds
1 tbsp cacao powder
½ tsp vanilla extract
225g/8oz spinach

Method
Rinse the spinach well and drain.
Peel and de-stone the avocado.
Place all of the ingredients into a high-speed blender and add a little water it need be, so to make up to the level that will fill your glass.
Blend the ingredients until smooth. Enjoy immediately.

Chef's Note

Raw cacao contains nearly four times the antioxidant content of processed dark chocolate.

Macadamia Cauliflower Blast

Serves 1
302 calories

Ingredients
225g/8oz cauliflower
½ avocado
140g/4½oz courgette
1 tbsp macadamia
250ml/8½floz unsweetened almond milk
Water

Method
Rinse the cauliflower and roughly chop.
Rinse and roughly chop the courgette, leaving the skin and seeds intact.
Remove the peel and de-stone the avocado.
Add all of the ingredients into a high-speed blender and add a little water if necessary, so to fill the glass you are using.
Process the ingredients until smooth. Enjoy immediately.

Chef's Note
Macadamias are high in vitamin A, iron and protein and a tasty source of energy in a Keto diet.

Rhubarb And Ginger Smoothie

Serves 1
192 calories

Ingredients
250ml/8½floz unsweetened almond milk
½oz avocado
1 tsp ginger root
100g/3½oz rhubarb
1 tsp keto sweetener of your choice
1 tbsp goji berries
Water

Method
Rinse the rhubarb and roughly chop..
Prepare the ginger root by grating it into a high-speed blender.
Add all of the ingredients to the ginger and top up with a little water if needed, so to fill the glass you are using. Blend the ingredients until smooth. Enjoy immediately.

Chef's Note
Goji berries have higher levels of antioxidants than nearly all other superfoods and a great energy source.

Super Fuel Smoothie

Serves 1
276 calories

Ingredients
200g/7oz kale
½ avocado
1 tbsp hemp seeds
3-4 fennel seeds
250ml/8½floz unsweetened almond milk
Water
Ice

Method
Rinse the kale and remove any thick stems.
Peel the avocado and remove the stone.
Crush the fennel seeds a little.
Add all of the ingredients into a high-speed blender and add a little water if need be, so the level will fill the glass you are using,
Blend until smooth. Enjoy immediately with plenty of ice.

Chef's Note
Make sure you use unsweetened almond milk when making Keto smoothies.

Watercress Cream Smoothie

Serves 1
170 calories

Ingredients
225g/8oz watercress
75g/3oz cucumber

2 tbsp single cream
250ml/8½floz unsweetened almond milk
1 tbsp ground almonds
Water

Method
Rinse the watercress and drain well.
Rinse and roughly chop the cucumber, leaving the skin and seeds intact.
Add all of the ingredients into a high-speed blender and add a little water so the level will fill the glass you are using.
Process the ingredients until smooth. Enjoy immediately.

Chef's Note
The added ground almonds create more creaminess and brings energy and fibre to this smoothie.

Spice Energiser
Serves 1
162 calories

Ingredients
120ml/4floz coconut water
175g/6oz aubergine
1 orange or red bell pepper
1 tsp turmeric
1/2 tsp cumin
1 tbsp cashew nuts

Water

Method
Wash the aubergine and roughly chop.
Wash and remove the seeds from the pepper and roughly chop.
Roughly chop the cashews.
Add all of the ingredients into a high-speed blender and add a little water if needed so the level will fill the glass you are using.
Blend the ingredients until smooth. Enjoy immediately.

Chef's Note
Try soaking the cashew nuts in water overnight to create an even creamier drink.

Coconut Spinach Smoothie
Serves 1
375 calories

Ingredients
225g/8oz spinach
2 tbsp coconut cream
½ avocado
1 tbsp hemp seeds
200ml/7floz coconut water
Water

Method
Rinse the spinach well and drain.

Remove the skin and stone from the avocado.

Add all of the ingredients into a high-speed blender and add a little water if necessary so it comes to a level that will fill the glass you are using.

Process the ingredients until smooth. Enjoy immediately.

Chef's Note
Make sure you use the full fat version of coconut mik to get the best energy hit.

Exotic Sumac Boost

Serves 1
279 calories

Ingredients
200g/7oz cauliflower
1 tsp sumac
1 tbsp flaxseed
250ml/8 ½floz unsweetened almond milk
100g/3½oz avocado
Water

Method
Rinse the cauliflower and cut into florets.
Peel and stone the avocado.
Add all of the ingredients into a high-speed blender and add a little water if need be, to make up to the level to fill the glass you are using.

Process the ingredients until smooth. Enjoy immediately.

Chef's Note
Sumac is a widely used spice, tasting of mild peppery, lemon. It is considered a great anti-inflammatory ingredient.

Green Tea Cool Fuel

Serves 1
188 calories

Ingredients
250ml/8½floz green tea, cooled
½ avocado
3 tbsp full fat Greek yoghurt
200g/7oz cucumber
1 tsp matcha powder
2 tsp mint leaves
Water

Method
Wash and roughly chop the cucumber, leaving the seeds and skin intact.
Rinse and drain the mint leaves.
Add all of the ingredients into a high-speed blender and add a little more water if you want a longer drink.
Process the ingredients until everything is really smooth. Serve immediately.

Matcha powder is full of vitamin C, selenium, zinc and magnesium.

Fuel Stop Smoothie

Serves 1
340 calories

Ingredients
½ avocado
1 tsp vanilla extract
2 tbsp macadamia
2 tbsp full fat Greek yoghurt
200ml/7floz coconut milk
water

Method
Peel and stone the avocado.
Chop the macadamia nuts a little to help with blending.
Add all of the ingredients into a high-speed blender and add a little water if needed, so the level will fill the glass you are using.
Process the ingredients until smooth.
Enjoy immediately.

Chef's Note
This smoothie is full of good fats and low carbohydrates. It's an excellent choice for when you feel you need a hit of energy but don't fancy lots of green veg!

Spiced Green Smoothie

Serves 1
179 calories

Ingredients
75g/3oz kale
2 celery stalks
½ tsp spirulina
1 pinch ground cinnamon
1 tsp grated ginger root
175ml/6oz unsweetened almond milk
3 tbsp full fat Greek Yoghurt
Water

Method
Rinse the kale and the celery. Chop the celery and remove the thick stems from the kale.
Add all the ingredients to a high-speed blender. Top with a little water so the level will the glass you are using,
Process the ingredients until smooth. Enjoy immediately.

Chef's Note
Spirulina is a great source of nutrients including vitamins B, C, D, A and E and worth stocking for Keto plans.

Hemp & Sweet Pepper Smoothie

Serves 1
320 calories

Ingredients
225g/8oz spinach
60g/2oz yellow or orange pepper
1 stalk celery
1 tbsp hemp seeds
½ avocado
175ml/6oz unsweetened almond milk
2 tbsp full fat Greek Yoghurt
½ tsp oregano leaves
Water

Method
Rinse the spinach, oregano, pepper and celery.
De-seed the pepper. Peel & de-stone the avocado.
Rinse and roughly chop the celery.
Add all of the ingredients to a high-speed blender and top up with water if necessary so the level will fill the glass you are using,
Process until smooth. Enjoy immediately.

Chef's Note
Make sure you use full fat Greek yoghurts when preparing keto smoothies,

Cucumber & Dill Nutter

Serves 1
254 calories

Ingredients
5 sprigs fresh dill
300g/11oz cucumber
250ml/8½floz unsweetened almond milk
½ avocado
10 raw pistachio nuts
Water
Ice cubes

Method
Roughly chop the cucumber, leaving the skin and seeds intact.
Wash the dill and drain well.
Peel & de-stone the avocado.
Add all of the ingredients to a high speed blender and top up with a little water if need be, so to fill the glass you will be using.
Blend the ingredients until really smooth. Enjoy immediately.

Chef's Note
Pistachios are a good source of fibre, protein, and heart-healthy fats.

Veg Head

Serves 1
309 calories

Ingredients
250ml/8½floz unsweetened almond milk
225g/8oz spinach
175g/6oz tomatoes
150g/5oz courgette
½ avocado
1 tbsp hemp seeds
water

Method
Rinse the spinach, tomatoes & courgettes and roughly chop.
Peel and de-stone the avocado.
Add all of the ingredients to a high-speed blender, topping up with water if needed, so you can fill the glass you are using,
Process the ingredients until really smooth. Enjoy immediately.

Chef's Note
Blender Tip....if you sometimes find your ingredients won't all fit in your cup under the max line. Try blending some together first to make room for the other ingredients.

Veggie Hazelnut Smoothie

Serves 1
392 calories

Ingredients
½ avocado
150g/5oz cucumber
1 tbsp hazelnuts
125g/4oz tomatoes
75g/3oz kale
1 tbsp lemon juice
250ml/8½floz unsweetened almond milk
Water

Method
Rinse the kale and remove any tough stems.
Peel and de-stone the avocado.
Wash and roughly chop the cucumber, keeping the skin and seeds intact.
Wash the tomatoes and roughly chop.
Add all of the ingredients to a high-speed blender, topping up with a little water if you need to so you can fill the glass you will be using.
Blend the ingredients together until really smooth. Enjoy immediately.

Chef's Note
Hazelnuts are a rich source of dietary fibre, manganese, vitamin B1, and the essential fatty acid omega-3.

Double Almond Boost

Serves 1
389 calories

Ingredients
75g/3oz cucumber
50g/2oz avocado
1 tbsp almond butter
2cm/1inch piece fresh root ginger
1 tsp ground cinnamon
225g/8oz spinach
200ml/7floz unsweetened almond milk
Water

Method
Rinse the spinach & cucumber and roughly chop.
Peel and de-stone the avocado.
Peel and grate the ginger.
Add all the ingredients to a high-speed blender and top with a little water if needed, so you can fill the glass you are going to use.
Blend the ingredients until smooth. Enjoy immediately.

Chef's Note
Almond butter is a source of vitamin E, copper, magnesium, and high quality protein.

Red Devil Boost

Serves 1

288 calories

Ingredients
200g/7oz tomato
60g/2oz red pepper
75g/3oz romaine lettuce
½ avocado
½ tsp ground cinnamon
Pinch of cayenne pepper
1 tbsp Brazil nuts
200ml/7oz coconut water
Water

Method
Rinse the tomato, pepper and lettuce. Core and roughly chop the pepper.
Peel and de-stone the avocado.
Chop the Brazil nuts a little to help blending.
Add all of the ingredients to a high-speed blender and top up with water if need be, so the level will fill the glass you are using.
Process the ingredients until smooth. Enjoy immediately.

Chef's Note
Tomatoes are an excellent source of vitamin C and add a natural sweetness to keto dishes.

Get Up Thyme

Serves 1

215 calories

Ingredients
150g/5oz cucumber
1 tbsp fresh thyme
225g/8oz spinach
1 tbsp lemon juice
½ avocado
1 tbsp ground almonds
250ml/8½floz coconut water
Water

Method
Rinse the cucumber, thyme and spinach.
Roughly chop the cucumber, keeping the skin and seeds intact..
Peel and de-stone the avocado.
Add all of the ingredients to a high-speed blender and top with a little water if needed, so it will fill the glass you are using.
Blend the ingredients until smooth. Enjoy immediately.

Chef's Note
Thyme is rich in many vital vitamins, including Vitamin C, B 12, K and A.

Mean Green Machine
Serves 1
273 calories

Ingredients

50g/2oz broccoli
75g/3oz kale
225g/8oz spinach
½ avocado
1 tbsp lemon juice
1 tsp chia seeds
1 tsp matcha powder
200ml/7floz coconut water
Water

Method

Wash the broccoli, kale and spinach. Cut any thick stems off the kale.
Peel and de-stone the avocado.
Put all of the ingredients into a high-speed blender and add a little water if needed, so to fill the glass you are using.
Process the ingredients until smooth. Enjoy immediately.

Chef's Note

This smoothie contains a huge spectrum of vitamins and minerals and is a good meal replacement.

Endive Energy

Serves 1
348 calories

Ingredients

½ avocado
150g/5oz endive
225g/8oz spinach
1 celery stalk
250ml/8½floz unsweetened almond milk
1 tbsp flat leaf parsley
Water

Method
Wash the endive, parsley and spinach and drain well.
Peel and de-stone the avocado.
Add all of the ingredients to a high-speed blender and add a little water if needed, to make up to the level that will fill the glass you are using.
Process the ingredients until smooth. Enjoy immediately.

Chef's Note
Almond milk is high in energy, proteins, lipids and fibre.

Cashew Butter & Spinach Smoothie
Serves 1
396 calories

Ingredients
1 tbsp cashew butter
1 tbsp cashews
225g/8oz spinach
100g/3½oz avocado
250ml coconut water

Ice cubes

Method
Rinse the spinach well and drain.
Peel and de-stone the avocado.
Add all the ingredients to a high-speed blender and add a little water if need be, so to fill the glass you are using.
Blend the ingredients until smooth. Enjoy immediately.

Chef's Note
Vary the nuts and nut butter to suit your own taste, they will all provide you with a great boost of energy.

Deconstructed Pesto Smoothie

Serves 1
266 calories

Ingredients
150g/5oz rocket leaves
½ avocado
1 tbsp pine nuts
250ml/8½floz unsweetened almond milk
1 garlic clove
1 tbsp parmesan cheese
Water

Method
Wash the rocket and drain well.
Crush the pine nuts a little and crush the garlic clove.

Add all of the ingredients to a high-speed blender and top up with a little water if need be, so it will fill the glass you are using.

Process the ingredients until smooth. Enjoy immediately.

Chef's Note
This is a great smoothie if you need a calcium boost, your bones and teeth will thank you for it!

Pumpkin Seed Rush

Serves 1
421 calories

Ingredients
½ avocado
2 tbsp pumpkin seeds
125g/4oz kale
125g/4oz cucumber
250ml/8½floz unsweetened almond milk
Water

Method
Peel and remove the stone in the avocado.
Wash and drain the kale, removing any thick stems.
Rinse and roughly chop the cucumber, keeping the skin and seeds intact.
Add all of the ingredients to a high-speed blender and add a little water if need be, so the level will fill the glass you are using.

Process the ingredients until smooth. Enjoy immediately.

Chef's Note
You could also use other milk as an alternative, but choose ones that are low in sugar and carbohydrates..

Herb Bullet

Serves 1
358 calories

Ingredients
½ avocado
225g/8oz spinach
2 tbsp walnuts
200ml/7floz bone broth
1 tbsp flat leaf parsley
1 tbsp chives
1 tbsp thyme leaves
1 tsp coconut oil

Method
Rinse the spinach and drain.
Rinse and drain the herbs.
Add all of the ingredients to a high-speed blender.
Blend until everything is smooth.
Enjoy immediately.

Chef's Note

This savoury smoothie is full of flavour and a great hit of nutrition for a keto plan.

Super Green Shot

Serves 1
245 calories

Ingredients
1 tsp spirulina
1 tbsp hemp seed
125g/4oz broccoli
125g/4oz kale
125g/green cabbage
120ml/4floz bone broth

Method
Wash and roughly cut the cabbage, kale and broccoli, removing any tough stems or stalks.
Add everything to a high-speed blender. This is a really short drink, so don't add any extra water. You could even serve in shot glasses.
Blend the ingredients until really smooth. Enjoy immediately.

Chef's Note
Bone broth has great healing properties and a wealth of protein building blocks.

Nutty Lemon Lift

Serves 1
288 calories

Ingredients
1 tbsp brazil nuts
200g/7oz courgette
2 tbsp full fat Greek Yoghurt
200ml/7floz unsweetened almond milk
1 tsp lemon verbena leaves
1 lemon
Pinch ground cardamom
Water

Method
Wash and roughly chop the courgette, leaving the skin and seeds intact.
Wash and drain the lemon verbena leaves.
Roughly chop the brazil nuts, to help the blending.
Add all of the ingredients to a high-speed blender and add a little more water if need be so the level will fill the glass you are using.
Process until smooth and enjoy immediately.

Chef's Note
Brazil nuts are a source of selenium and will give both your mood and your energy a lift.

Rhubarb & Custard Energiser

Serves 1
304 calories

Ingredients

100g/3½oz rhubarb
½ avocado
200ml/7floz unsweetened almond milk
2 tbsp pecan nuts
½ tsp nutmeg
1 tsp vanilla extract
2 tbsp single cream
Water

Method

Wash and roughly chop the rhubarb.
Remove the peel and de-stone the avocado.
Roughly chop the pecans a little.
Add all of the ingredients to a high-speed blender and top up with water if need be, to enable you to fill the glass you are using.
Blend the ingredients well, until really smooth. Enjoy immediately.

Chef's Note

These flavours are similar to this classic combo and the added pecans provide protein to help energise you.

Flax Fuse

Serves 1
286 calories

Ingredients
2 tbsp flaxseeds
½ avocado
125g/4oz cucumber
200ml/7floz coconut water
Water
Ice cubes

Method
Remove the peel and de-stone the avocado.
Wash and roughly chop the cucumber, keeping the skin and seeds intact.
Add all of the ingredients to a high-speed blender, adding water if need be to the level that will fill the glass you are using.
Process the ingredients until really smooth. Enjoy immediately with ice for an extra cold drink.

Chef's Note
Flaxseeds are a source of energy and lignans, compounds thought to reduce risk of developing certain cancers.

Butter Boost Smoothie

Serves 1

189 calories

Ingredients
150g/5oz frozen blueberries
1 tbsp almond butter
1 tbsp tahini
300ml/10½ floz coconut water
Ice

Method
Don't defrost the blueberries - use them straight from the freezer.
Add all of the ingredients to a high-speed blender, except the ice.
Blend the ingredients until smooth.
Top with a large handful of ice and enjoy this slushie smoothie immediately.

Chef's Note
Berries can be used in a Keto plan and they are full of health boosting flavanoids, but only consume in moderation.

Ginger Punch

Serves 1
339 calories

Ingredients
200g/7oz cucumber
2 tsp ginger root, grated

½ avocado
1 tbsp macadamia nuts
200ml/7floz hemp milk
Water

Method
Wash and roughly chop the cucumber, keeping the skin and seeds intact.
Remove the peel and de-stone the avocado.
Prepare the ginger and add to a high-speed blender.
Add all of the other ingredients to the blender and top with a little water if needed, to make the level up to be able to fill your glass.
Process the ingredients until smooth. Enjoy immediately.

Chef's Note
Ginger is known for it's wonderful anti-inflammatory properties and is a great addition to a keto diet.

Nutty Green Boost
Serves 1
406 calories

Ingredients
225g/8oz spinach
½ avocado
1 tbsp chopped fresh lemon verbena
2tbsp almond butter
200ml/7floz unsweetened almond milk

Water

Method
Rinse the spinach.
Peel and de-stone the avocado.
Rinse and dry the lemon verbena leaves.
Add all of the ingredients into a high-speed blender and top up with a little water if need be so it will fill the glass you are using.
Process the ingredients until smooth. Enjoy immediately.

Chef's Note
Almonds are a great source of protein and magnesium and will help keep you feeling fuller for longer.

Full Keto Smoothies

Bulletproof Coffee Smoothie
Serves 1
402 calories

Ingredients
250ml/8½floz coffee
1 tbsp coconut oil, melted
1 tbsp butter, melted
1 tsp vanilla extract
1/2 tsp cinnamon
4 tbsp whipping cream
ice to serve

Method

Place all of the ingredients, apart from the ice, into a high-speed blender.

Blend the ingredients until the whipping cream starts to thicken and froth.

Pour into a glass and top with plenty of ice.

Chef's Note

Bulletproof coffee is a Keto friendly energy boosting drink and this iced smoothie version is a great start to a summer's morning.

Chocomint Smoothie

Serves 1
145 calories

Ingredients

1 tbsp single cream
1 tbsp raw cacao powder
2 tbsp mint leaves
250m/8½floz coconut water
Water

Method

Wash and drain the mint leaves (you could use any variety of mint leaves for this recipe; the chocolate mint leaf goes really well).

Place the cream, cacao powder, mint and coconut water into a high-speed blender.

Process the ingredients until all of the ingredients are really smooth.
Serve in a glass with an extra sprinkle of cacao powder and an optional spoonful of thick, whipped cream.

Chef's Note
Try with any unsweetened Keto friendly milk for this recipe.

Protein Berry Blast

Serves 1
209 calories

Ingredients
175g/6oz strawberries
1 tbsp hemp seed
1 tbsp sunflower seeds
250ml/8½ floz unsweetened almond milk
Water

Method
Rinse and hull the strawberries. Roughly chop.
Add all of the ingredients to a high-speed blender and top with a little water if need be, so you can fill the glass you are using.
Blend the ingredients until smooth. Serve immediately.

Chef's Note
Protein is vital to muscle growth and tissue repair and is found in hemp and sunflower seeds.

Strawberries & Cream

Serves 1
259 calories

Ingredients
175g/6oz strawberries
3 tbsp single cream
200ml/7floz unsweetened almond milk
1 tsp vanilla extract
A few mint leaves to serve
Ice to serve

Method
Rinse and hull the strawberries and roughly chop.
Place all of the ingredients into a high-speed blender and top up with water if need be, so you can fill the glass you are using.
Blend the ingredients until really smooth.
Enjoy immediately with mint leaves and plenty of ice.

Chef's Note
Strawberries can be eaten in moderation when you have balanced your Keto diet, just be sure to not over do them!

Middle Eastern Promise

Serves 1
387 calories

Ingredients
200g/7oz blackberries
50g/2oz blueberries
1 tbsp brazil nuts
100ml/3½oz full fat Greek yogurt
200ml/7floz almond milk
Water

Method
Rinse and drain the blackberries and blueberries,
Add all of the ingredients to a high-speed blender and
top up with a little water if needed, so the level will fill
the glass you are using.
Blend the ingredients until smooth. Enjoy immediately.

Chef's Note
Blackberries are a great source of manganese.

Almond & Chia Smoothie

Serves 1
317 calories

Ingredients
½ avocado
2 tbsp almond butter
250ml/ 8½floz unsweetened almond milk
1 tbsp chia seeds
Water

Method
Remove the peel and de-stone the avocado.

Place the avocado flesh, almond butter, almond milk and chia seeds into a high speed blender, adding a little more water if necessary so you can fill the glass you are using.

Process the ingredients until really smooth.

Serve immediately.

Chef's Note
Almonds can add magnesium to your diet, which promotes blood flow to the heart.

Coconut Berry Blast
238 calories

Serves 1

Ingredients
150g/5oz mixed berries (blueberries, raspberries or blackberries)

250ml/8½floz coconut water

1 tbsp coconut cream

15g/½oz pumpkin seeds

Water

Method
Wash and drain the berries.

Add the coconut water, coconut cream and pumpkin seeds to a high-speed blender and top up with water if needed, so you can fill the glass you are using.

Blend the ingredients until they are smooth.
Serve immediately.

Chef's Note
Use the thick coconut cream block here to add with the milk as it will bring a lovely depth of coconut flavour to this drink.

Coffee & Cinnamon Boost

Serves 1
126 calories

Ingredients
½ tsp cinnamon
3 tbsp single cream
200ml/7floz coffee, cooled
½ tsp vanilla
Ice

Method
Add all of the ingredients into a high-speed blender and add a handful of ice.
Process until the ingredients are well mixed and the ice has broken down.
Serve this iced smoothie immediately.

Chef's Note
Experiment with more cinnamon and even some nutmeg too, for a warmer, spicier taste.

Raspberry & White Chocolate Cooler

Serves 1
222 calories

Ingredients

200g/7oz raspberries
1 tsp cocoa butter
½ tsp coconut oil, melted
200ml/7floz unsweetened almond milk
1 tsp vanilla extract
Ice

Method

Rinse the raspberries well.
Add all of the ingredients to a high-speed blender.
apart from the ice.
Blend the ingredients until smooth.
Add a handful of ice to the cooler and serve immediately,

Chef's Note

Try and find raw cocoa butter as it has a higher level of nutrients.

Gingerbread Fat Bomb Smoothie

Serves 1
220 calories

Ingredients

1 tsp ground ginger
1 tsp ground cinnamon
1 tbsp almond flour
1 tbsp almond butter
½ tsp stevia/Keto sweetener
200ml/7oz coconut milk
2 tbsp melted butter
1 tbsp lemon juice

Method
Put all of the ingredients into a high-speed blender. Process until everything is well combined and smooth. Add a little more stevia/sweetener to taste and serve immediately.

Chef's Note
This high energy and high fat smoothie is perfect for those following a Keto diet.

Lemon Cheesecake Smoothie
Serves 1
182 calories

Ingredients
1 lemon, zest and juice
4 tbsp cream cheese
200ml/7floz unsweetened almond milk
½ tsp ground ginger
Water

Method

Wash the lemon and zest it. Squeeze all of the juice out (try rolling this on the worktop with a firm hand beforehand so the juice is easier to squeeze).

Add all of the ingredients to a high-speed blender, topping up with a little water if needed, so you can fill the glass you are using.

Blend the ingredients until smooth.

Enjoy immediately.

Chef's Note

Lemons are full of vitamin C and a great anti-oxidant.

Gooseberry Bomb

Serves 1
345 calories

Ingredients

175g/6oz gooseberries
½ avocado
1 tbsp mint leaves
1 tbsp chia seeds
2 tbsp single cream
250ml/8 floz unsweetened almond milk
1 tbsp chia seeds
Water

Method

Rinse and drain the gooseberries, removing any stalks.
Peel and de-stone the avocado.

Add all of the ingredients to a high-speed blender, topping up with a little water if need be, so you can fill the glass you are using.
Blend until all of the ingredients are blended. Enjoy immediately.

Chef's Note
Gooseberries are a good source of vitamin C, manganese and dietary fibre.

Raspberry Salad Shake
Serves 1
288 calories

Ingredients
200g/7floz raspberries
125g/4oz rocket leaves
½ avocado
1 tsp oregano leaves
200ml/7floz unsweetened almond milk
Water

Method
Rinse the raspberries and drain.
Peel and de-stone the avocado.
Wash and drain the rocket and oregano.
Add all of the ingredients to a high-speed blender and add a little water if need be, so the level will fill the glass you are using.
Blend until smooth. Enjoy immediately.

Chef's Note
The ellagic acid in raspberries is thought to be a useful compound in reducing the risk of developing some cancers.

Part 2

85

Introduction

This book has a wide selection of smoothie recipes that you can enjoy any time of the day.

Smoothies are very easy to make. You only need a liquid base (milk, yogurt, fruit juice, or water), some fruits or vegetables, a bit of seeds or nuts if desired, and of course a good blender.

Smoothies are very versatile. You can mix and match some of the ingredients or add more depending on your taste and health requirement. For some people that can't take dairies, there are other options that are equally delicious and nutritious like soy-based milk or yogurt, rice milk, almond milk, and coconut milk.

They are also fun to make because you can add any ingredient that you desire. Even your kids can help you in making them because the process is very easy and simple, you just need to put everything in your blender and there you have it – a refreshing drink in less than 5 minutes!

Smoothies are for everyone to enjoy. By drinking a glass of healthy smoothie a day can ensure that you are getting enough vitamins and minerals that your body needs. It is also a good way of using your fruits and vegetables since they are highly perishable. Strawberries, bananas, and milk are common smoothie ingredients that are easily found in supermarkets. Feel free to browse on the recipes on this book and for sure you can whip something good out of these simple yet delicious ingredients.

Read on and I hope you'll enjoy all the recipes in this book.

Mango Orange And Strawberry Smoothie

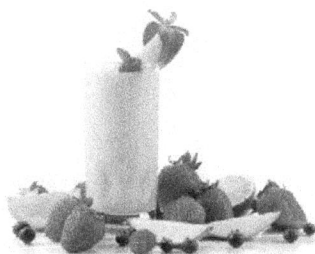

Preparation Time: 5 minutes**Yield:** 2 servings

Ingredients

1 cup mango
1/2 cup seedless orange segments
1/4 cup strawberries
1 cup low-fat milk

6 ice cubes

Method

1. Peel both the mango and the orange and cut them into small pieces.
2. Hull the strawberries and also cut them into small pieces.
3. Put all fruits in the blender along with the milk and ice cubes.
4. Blend until smooth and pour into 2 serving glasses.
5. Serve immediately and enjoy.

Nutritional Information:
Energy – 137 kcal, Fat – 2.9 g, Carbs - 25 g, Protein – 5.2g, Sodium – 59 mg

Avocado Almond And Yogurt Smoothie

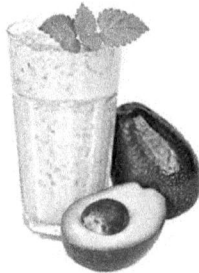

Preparation Time: 5 minutes **Yield:** 4 servings

Ingredients

1 medium avocado
2 ½ cups almond milk
1 cup vanilla-flavored yogurt
1 Tbsp. honey
1 cup ice cubes

Method
1. Remove and discard pit from avocado. Cut into small pieces and place into the blender along with the almond milk, yogurt, honey, and ice cubes.
2. Blend until smooth then transfer into 3 chilled tall glasses.
3. Serve immediately and enjoy.

Nutritional Information:

Energy – 181 kcal, Fat – 12.1 g, Carbs - 13.6 g, Protein – 5.1g, Sodium – 140 mg

Blackberry Strawberry And Coconut Smoothie

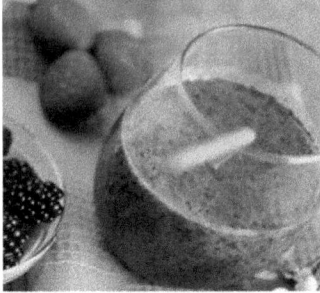

Preparation Time: 5 minutes**Yield:** 2 servings

Ingredients

1/2 cup frozen blackberries
1/2 cup frozen strawberries
1 cup coconut water
1/4 cup coconut milk
1 Tbsp. honey

Method
1. Place the blackberries, strawberries, coconut water, coconut milk, and honey in a blender. Process until smooth and combined well.
2. Divide smoothie among 2 chilled glasses.
3. Serve with a straw and garnish with berries, if desired.

Nutritional Information:

Energy – 151 kcal, Fat – 7.7 g, Carbs - 21.0 g, Protein – 2.3 g, Sodium – 132 mg

V Blueberry Banana And Ricotta Smoothie

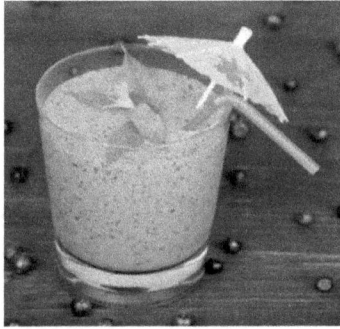

Preparation Time: 5 minutes**Yield:** 2 servings

Ingredients

1 medium frozen banana, sliced
1 cup frozen blueberries
1 cup skim milk
1/4 cup ricotta cheese
fresh mint sprigs

Method

1. Combine the banana, blueberries, skim milk, and ricotta cheese in a blender. Process until it becomes smooth.
2. Pour mixture into two chilled glasses. Garnish with fresh mint sprigs.
3. Serve and enjoy.

Nutritional Information:

Energy – 182 kcal, Fat – 2.9 g, Carbs - 31.6 g, Protein – 8.7 g, Sodium – 105 mg

Spiced Raspberry Yogurt And Soy Smoothie

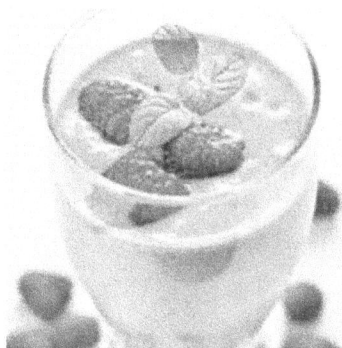

Preparation Time: 5 minutes **Yield:** 2 servings

Ingredients

1 cup frozen raspberries

6 oz. Greek yogurt (plain or vanilla)
1 cup soy milk
1/4 teaspoon cinnamon
1/4 teaspoon ground nutmeg
fresh mint sprig

Method

1. Place the raspberries, yogurt, soy milk, cinnamon, and nutmeg in a blender. Process until smooth and creamy.
2. Divide smoothie in 2 chilled glasses. Garnish with some raspberries and mint sprig, if desired.
3. Serve and enjoy.

Nutritional Information:

Energy – 161 kcal, Fat – 3.7 g, Carbs - 21.4 g, Protein – 9.6 g, Sodium – 123 mg

Almond Cherry And Banana Smoothie With Hemp Seeds

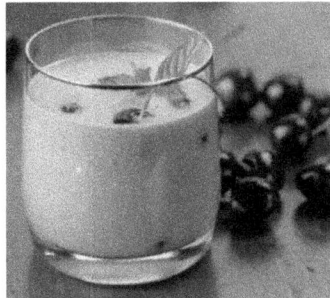

Preparation Time: 5 minutes**Yield:** 2 servings

Ingredients

1 cup frozen cherries, pitted
1 medium frozen banana, sliced
1 ½ cups almond milk
2 tsp. hemp seeds
fresh mint sprigs

Method
1. Combine the cherries, banana, almond milk, and hemp seeds in a blender. Process until it becomes smooth.
2. Pour smoothie in 2 chilled glasses. Garnish with some cherries and mint sprigs, if desired.
3. Serve and enjoy.

Nutritional Information:
Energy – 146 kcal, Fat – 3.8 g, Carbs - 25.5 g, Protein – 3.1 g, Sodium – 113 mg

Banana Cottage Cheese And Vanilla Smoothie

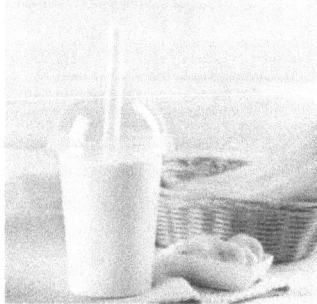

Preparation Time: 5 minutes**Yield:** 2 servings

Ingredients

2 medium frozen bananas, sliced
1/2 cup cottage cheese
1 1/2 cups almond milk, unsweetened
1 tsp. honey

Method
1. Place the banana, cottage cheese, almond milk, and honey ice in a blender. Process until smooth and creamy.
2. Pour and divide among 2 chilled glasses.
3. Serve immediately and enjoy.

Nutritional Information:

Energy – 189 kcal, Fat – 3.4 g, Carbs - 32.6 g, Protein – 9.8 g, Sodium – 143 mg

Banana Blueberries And Soy Smoothie With Flax

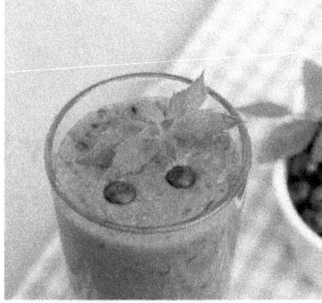

Preparation Time: 5 minutes **Yield:** 2 servings

Ingredients

1 medium frozen banana, sliced
1 cup frozen blueberries
1/2 cup organic soy milk
1/2 cup soy yogurt
1 Tbsp. flaxseeds
fresh mint sprigs

Method
1. Place the banana, blueberries, soy milk, soy yogurt, and flaxseeds in a blender. Process until smooth and creamy.
2. Pour smoothie in 2 chilled glasses. Garnish with some blueberries and fresh mint sprig, if desired.

3. Serve and enjoy.

Nutritional Information:
Energy – 193 kcal, Fat – 4.1 g, Carbs - 35.1 g, Protein – 6.3 g, Sodium – 38 mg

Grape Kiwi And Blueberry Smoothie

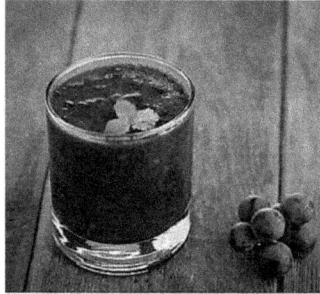

Preparation Time: 5 minutes**Yield:** 2 servings

Ingredients

1 cup of seedless grapes
2 medium kiwi fruit (peeled and cut into small pieces)
1 cup blueberries
1 cup of crushed ice
fresh mint sprig

Method

1. Place the grapes, kiwi, and blueberries in a blender. Process until smooth. Add the ice and then blend again for 15 seconds.
2. Pour and divide among 2 chilled glasses. Garnish with mint sprig, if desired.
3. Serve and enjoy.

Nutritional Information:

Energy – 119 kcal, Fat – 0.8 g, Carbs - 29.5 g, Protein – 1.7 g, Sodium – 4 mg

Banana Kiwi And Green Tea Smoothie

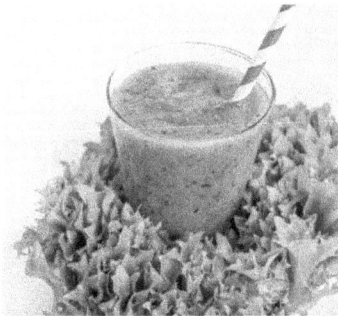

Preparation Time: 5 minutes**Yield:** 3 servings

Ingredients

2 medium frozen bananas, sliced
2 medium kiwi fruit, cubed
1 cup of kale, torn
1 ½ cup of freshly brewed green tea
1 cup of crushed ice

Method
1. Combine the banana, kiwi, kale, green tea, and crushed ice in a blender.
2. Blend everything together until smooth.
3. Pour into two glasses.
4. Serve immediately.

Nutritional Information:
Energy – 112 kcal, Fat – 0.5 g, Carbs - 27.7 g, Protein – 2.7 g, Sodium – 12 mg

Lychee Melon And Vanilla Smoothie

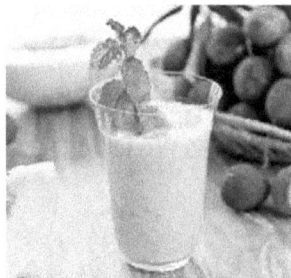

Preparation Time: 5 minutes**Yield:** 3 servings

Ingredients

1 cup lychees, peeled and pitted
1 cup rock melon, peeled, deseeded, and diced
1 cup low-fat milk
1 cup ice cubes
1/4 tsp. vanilla extract
fresh mint sprigs

Method
1. Combine the lychees, rock melon, low-fat milk, ice cubes, and vanilla extract in a blender. Process until it becomes smooth.
2. Pour and divide smoothie among 3 chilled glasses. Garnish fresh mint sprigs.
3. Serve immediately and enjoy.

Nutritional Information:
Energy – 150 kcal, Fat – 3.1 g, Carbs - 28.1 g, Protein – 5.5 g, Sodium – 71 mg

Banana Pear And Oat Smoothie

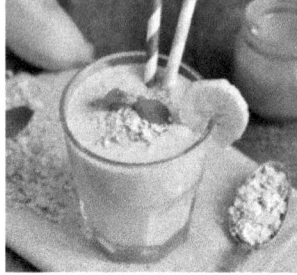

Preparation Time: 5 minutes**Yield:** 2 servings

Ingredients

1 medium frozen banana, sliced
2 cups almond milk, unsweetened
2 pear halves, peeled and cored
2 Tbsp. rolled oats
fresh mint sprigs

Method
1. Place the banana, almond milk, pear halves, and oats in a blender. Process until smooth and creamy.
2. Pour in 2 chilled glasses. Garnish with banana slices, some oats, and mint sprigs, if desired.
3. Serve immediately and enjoy.

Nutritional Information:

Energy – 142 kcal, Fat – 3.1 g, Carbs - 28.5 g, Protein – 2.6 g, Sodium – 152 mg

Creamy Mango-Apricot Smoothie With Cinnamon

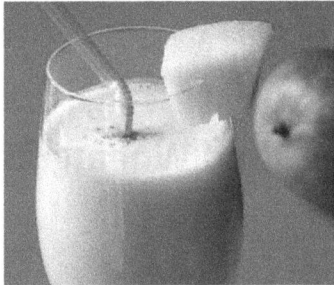

Preparation Time: 5 minutes**Yield:** 3 servings

Ingredients

1 cup mango, cut into cubes
4 apricots, pitted and halved
1 cup skim milk
1/2 cup vanilla yogurt
1/4 tsp. cinnamon, ground
1 cup crushed ice

Method

1. Combine the mango, apricots, skim milk, yogurt, cinnamon, and crushed ice in a blender. Process until it becomes smooth.
2. Pour and divide smoothie among 3 chilled glasses. Garnish with a small slice of mango and sprinkle with more cinnamon, if desired.
3. Serve immediately and enjoy.

Nutritional Information:

Energy – 172 kcal, Fat – 1.5 g, Carbs - 30.1 g, Protein – 9.1 g, Sodium – 110 mg

Mango Ginger And Wheatgrass Smoothie

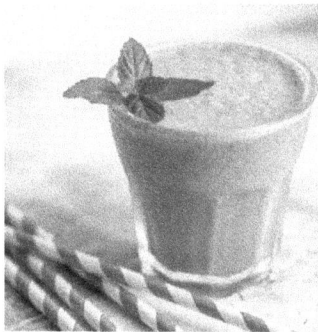

Preparation Time: 5 minutes**Yield:** 2 servings

Ingredients

1 ½ cups frozen mango
2 tsp. wheatgrass powder
2 Tbsp. lemon juice
1/4 tsp. ground ginger
1 cup coconut water
1 cup ice cubes

Method

1. Combine the mango, wheat grass powder, lemon juice, ginger, and coconut water in a blender. Process for 20 seconds or until blended well.
2. Add the ice cubes and blend again until it becomes smooth.
3. Pour and divide smoothie among 2 chilled glasses.
4. Serve and enjoy.

Nutritional Information:

Energy – 102 kcal, Fat – 0.8 g, Carbs - 23.5 g, Protein – 2.0 g, Sodium –130 mg

Mango And Orange Smoothie With Hemp Seed

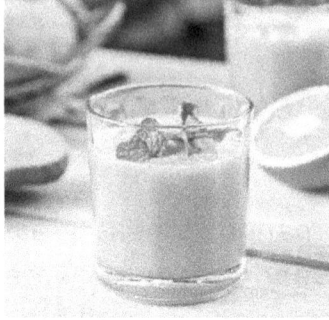

Preparation Time: 5 minutes**Yield:** 2 servings

Ingredients

1 cup mango, diced
1/2 cup of orange juice
1/2 cup Greek yogurt
2 tsp. hemp seeds
1 cup ice cubes
fresh mint sprigs

Method
1. Combine mango, orange juice, yogurt, hemp seeds, and ice cubes in your blender. Process until smooth.
2. Pour and divide smoothie among 2 chilled glasses.
3. Serve and enjoy.

Nutritional Information:

Energy – 142 kcal, Fat – 2.9 g, Carbs - 23.4 g, Protein – 5.8 g, Sodium – 44 mg

Mixed Berry Banana And Soy Smoothie

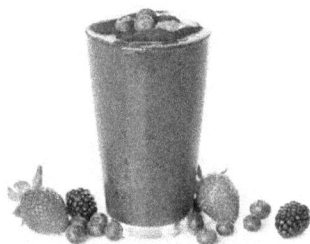

Preparation Time: 5 minutes**Yield:** 2 servings

Ingredients

1 cup frozen mixed berries
1 medium frozen banana, sliced
1 1/2 cups soy milk
fresh mint sprigs

Method

1. Place the mixed berries, banana, and soy milk in a high-speed blender. Process until smooth and creamy.

2. Pour in 2 chilled glasses. Garnish with a few blueberries and mint sprigs, if desired.
3. Serve and enjoy!

Nutritional Information:

Energy – 169 kcal, Fat – 2.7 g, Carbs - 32.2 g, Protein – 6.5 g, Sodium – 72 mg

Berry Kiwi And Lemon Smoothie

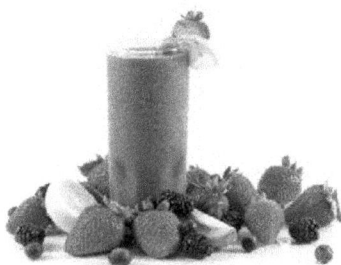

Preparation Time: 5 minutes**Yield:** 2 servings

Ingredients

1 cup frozen mixed berries
1 medium kiwi fruit, diced
1 cup skim milk
2 Tbsp. lemon juice
1 Tbsp. honey
1/2 cup crushed ice

lemon wedges
fresh mint sprigs

Method
1. Place the mixed berries, kiwi fruit, skim milk, lemon juice, honey, and ice in a blender. Process until it becomes smooth.
2. Pour and divide smoothie among 2 serving glasses. Garnish with lemon wedges and fresh mint sprig, if desired
3. Serve immediately and enjoy.

Nutritional Information:
Energy – 145 kcal, Fat – 0.6 g, Carbs - 31.0 g, Protein – 5.1 g, Sodium – 70 mg

Papaya Orange And Carrot Smoothie

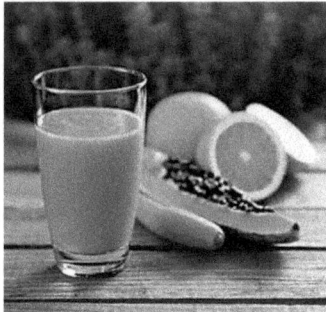

Preparation Time: 5 minutes**Yield:** 2 servings

Ingredients

1 ½ cups of papaya (cubed)
1 medium seedless orange (peeled and cut into segments)
1 cup carrot juice
1 cup of ice cubes

Method
1. Place the papaya, orange, carrot juice, and ice cubes in a high-speed blender. Process until it becomes smooth.
2. Pour mixture in 2 chilled glasses. Garnish with a slice of orange.
3. Serve immediately and enjoy.

Nutritional Information:
Energy – 100 kcal, Fat – 0.4 g, Carbs - 24.9 g, Protein – 1.6 g, Sodium – 47 mg

Papaya Banana And Pine Cooler

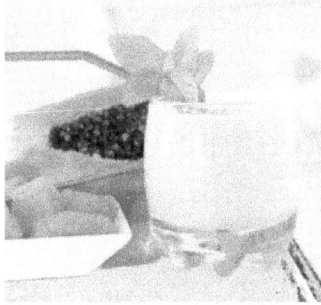

Preparation Time: 5 minutes**Yield:** 2 servings

Ingredients

1 cup papaya, cubed
1 medium frozen banana, sliced
1/2 cup pineapple tidbits
1/2 cup skim milk
2 Tbsp. coconut cream
1 cup crushed ice
fresh mint sprigs

Method
1. Place the papaya, banana, pineapple tidbits, skim milk, coconut cream, and crushed ice in a blender. Process until it becomes smooth.
2. Pour in 2 chilled glasses. Garnish with fresh mint sprigs.

3. Serve and enjoy!

Nutritional Information:

Energy – 161 kcal, Fat – 4.1 g, Carbs - 30.6 g, Protein – 3.6 g, Sodium – 42 mg

Raspberry Watermelon And Yogurt Smoothie

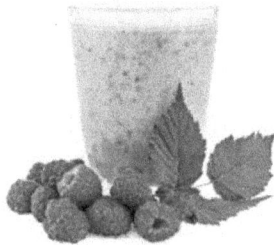

Preparation Time: 5 minutes**Yield:** 2 servings

Ingredients

1 cup frozen raspberries
1 cup watermelon
6 oz. Greek yogurt
1/2 cup low-fat milk
fresh mint sprigs

Method

1. Place the raspberries, watermelon, yogurt, and milk in a blender. Process until smooth.
2. Pour in 2 chilled glasses. Garnish with fresh mint sprigs.
3. Serve and enjoy. Recipe may be doubled if serving many people.

Nutritional Information:

Energy – 146 kcal, Fat – 2.8 g, Carbs - 22.0 g, Protein – 8.0 g, Sodium – 90 mg

Fig Banana And Cashew Smoothie

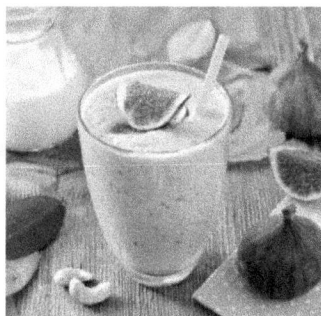

Preparation Time: 5 minutes **Yield:** 2 servings

Ingredients

2 medium figs, pulp only, cut into quarters

1 medium banana, sliced
2 Tbsp. cashew nuts
1 cup skim milk
1 cup ice cubes

Method
1. Combine the figs, banana, cashews, milk, and ice cubes in a blender. Process until it becomes smooth.
2. Pour and divide smoothie among 2 chilled glasses. Garnish with fig slices and serve with straw, if desired.
3. Enjoy.

Nutritional Information:
Energy – 182 kcal, Fat – 4.2 g, Carbs - 32.0 g, Protein – 7.0 g, Sodium – 67 mg

Red Currant Cranberry And Yogurt Delight

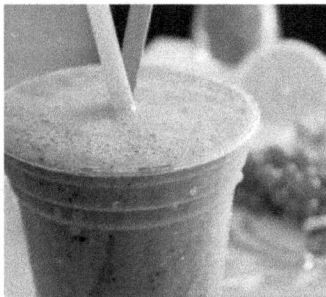

Preparation Time: 5 minutes **Yield:** 2 servings

Ingredients

1/2 cup of red currants
1/2 cup of cranberries
6 oz. low-fat yogurt
1 cup of ice cubes
2 tsp. agave nectar

Method
1. Combine the cranberries, red currants, low-fat yogurt, ice cubes, and agave nectar in a high-speed blender. Process until smooth.
2. Pour and divide among 2 chilled glasses.
3. Serve with straw and enjoy.

Nutritional Information:
Energy – 121 kcal, Fat – 1.1 g, Carbs - 20.4 g, Protein – 5.2 g, Sodium – 60 mg

Minty Strawberry And Yogurt Smoothie

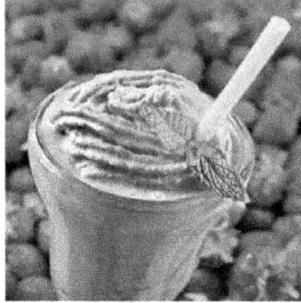

Preparation Time: 5 minutes**Yield:** 2 servings

Ingredients

1 cup frozen strawberries, hulled and halved
1 cup of skim milk
1/2 cup of Greek yogurt
1 Tbsp. peppermint syrup
fresh mint sprigs

Method
1. Combine the strawberries, milk, yogurt, and peppermint syrup in a blender. Process until it becomes smooth.
2. Pour and divide among 2 chilled glasses. Garnish with fresh mint sprigs.
3. Serve and enjoy.

Nutritional Information:

Energy – 117 kcal, Fat – 1.0 g, Carbs - 17.2 g, Protein – 8.0 g, Sodium – 109 mg

Pear Raspberry And Ricotta Smoothie

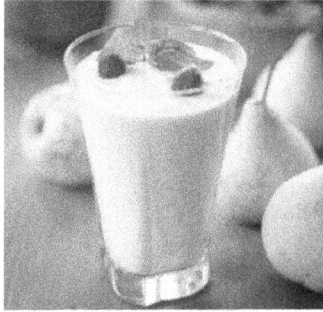

Preparation Time: 5 minutes **Yield:** 2 servings

Ingredients

1 cup frozen raspberries
1 medium pear, cored and diced
1 cup skim milk
1/2 cup ricotta cheese
fresh mint sprigs

Method

1. Combine the raspberries, pear, skim milk, and ricotta cheese in a blender. Process until it becomes smooth.
2. Pour and divide smoothie among 2 chilled glasses. Top with some raspberries and garnish with mint sprigs, if desired.
3. Serve immediately and enjoy.

Nutritional Information:

Energy – 203 kcal, Fat – 5.4 g, Carbs - 27.1 g, Protein – 12.1 g, Sodium – 144 mg

Yummy Strawberry Ricotta Cooler

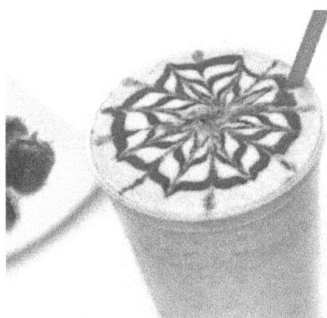

Preparation Time: 5 minutes **Yield:** 2 servings

Ingredients

1 cup frozen strawberries, halved
1 1/2 cup skim milk
1/3 cup ricotta cheese
2 Tbsp. strawberry syrup

Method
1. Combine the strawberries, ricotta cheese, and skim milk in a blender. Process until it becomes smooth.
2. Pour and divide mixture among 2 chilled glasses. Drizzle with strawberry syrup on top to decorate, if desired.
3. Serve and enjoy.

Nutritional Information:
Energy – 183 kcal, Fat – 2.7 g, Carbs - 29.1 g, Protein – 10.0 g, Sodium – 142 mg

Apple Banana And Peanut Butter Smoothie

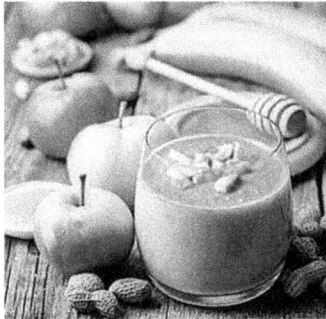

Preparation Time: 5 minutes **Yield:** 2 servings

Ingredients

1 medium frozen banana, sliced
1 medium apple, cored and diced
1 cup almond milk, unsweetened
1 Tbsp. peanut butter
1 cup ice cubes
chopped peanuts

Method
1. Combine the banana, apple, almond milk, peanut butter, and ice cubes in a high-speed blender. Process until smooth and creamy.
2. Pour and divide smoothie among 2 chilled glasses. Sprinkle with chopped peanuts.
3. Serve immediately and enjoy.

Nutritional Information:
Energy – 202 kcal, Fat – 9.5 g, Carbs - 28.1 g, Protein – 5.6 g, Sodium – 149 mg

Banana Strawberry And Flax Smoothie

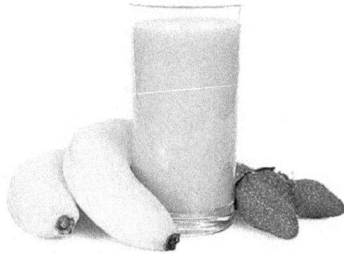

Preparation Time: 5 minutes**Yield:** 2 servings

Ingredients

1/2 cup low-fat milk
1/2 cup low-fat vanilla yogurt
1 medium frozen banana, sliced
1 cup frozen strawberries
1 Tbsp. flaxseeds

Method
1. Combine the milk, yogurt, banana, strawberries, and flaxseeds in a blender. Process until it becomes smooth.
2. Pour and divide smoothie among 2 chilled glasses.
3. Serve immediately and enjoy.

Nutritional Information:

Energy – 198 kcal, Fat – 3.5 g, Carbs - 34.3 g, Protein – 7.3 g, Sodium – 74 mg

Easy Mango Cheesecake Smoothie

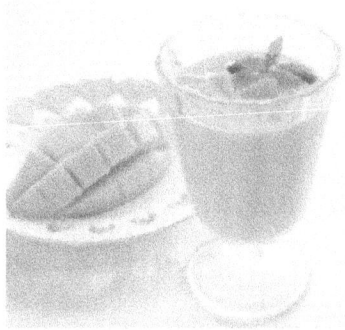

Preparation Time: 5 minutes**Yield:** 2 servings

Ingredients

1 cup mango, diced
1/4 cup mascarpone cheese
1 cup skim milk
2 Tbsp. crushed grahams
6 ice cubes

Method

1. Combine mango, mascarpone cheese, skim milk, grahams, and ice cubes in a blender. Process until it becomes smooth.
2. Pour and divide smoothie among 2 chilled glasses. Garnish with diced mangoes and mint sprigs, if desired.
3. Serve immediately and enjoy.

123

Nutritional Information:

Energy – 181 kcal, Fat – 5.1 g, Carbs - 25.6 g, Protein – 25.6 g, Sodium – 132 mg

Banana Strawberry Cereal And Yogurt Smoothie

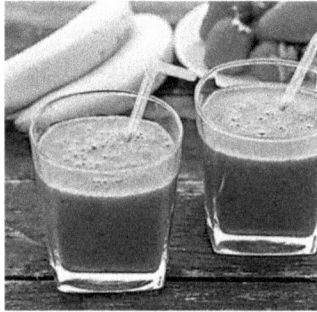

Preparation Time: 5 minutes**Yield:** 2 servings

Ingredients

1 medium frozen banana, sliced
1/2 cup frozen strawberries, hulled and halved
1 cup skim milk
6 oz. low-fat vanilla yogurt
2 Tbsp. granola

1 Tbsp. wheat germ

Method
1. Place banana, strawberries, milk, yogurt, granola, and wheat germ in a high-speed blender. Process until smooth and creamy.
2. Pour and divide among 2 chilled glasses.
3. Serve with straw and enjoy.

Nutritional Information:

Energy – 201 kcal, Fat – 5.4 g, Carbs - 38.1 g, Protein – 13.0 g, Sodium – 129 mg

Blackberry Almond And Oat Cooler

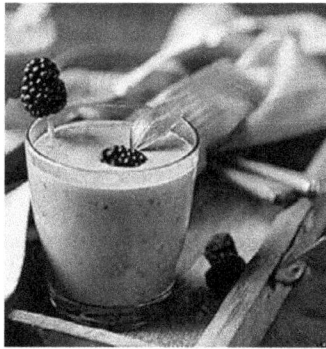

Preparation Time: 5 minutes**Yield:** 2 servings

Ingredients

1 cup frozen blackberries
1 cup almond milk
1/2 cup low-fat yogurt
2 Tbsp. rolled oats
2 tsp. honey
fresh mint sprigs

Method
1. Combine the blackberries, almond milk, yogurt, oats, and honey in a blender. Process until it becomes smooth.
2. Pour and divide smoothie among 2 chilled glasses. Top with some blackberries and mint sprigs, if desired.
3. Serve immediately and enjoy.

Nutritional Information:

Energy – 130 kcal, Fat – 2.7 g, Carbs - 21.0 g, Protein – 5.7 g, Sodium – 119 mg

Delightful Tofu Banana And Cinnamon Smoothie

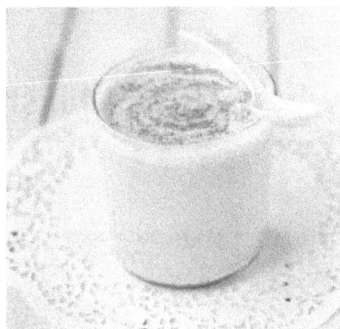

Preparation Time: 5 minutes**Yield:** 2 servings

Ingredients

1 medium frozen banana, sliced
1/2 cup silken tofu
1/2 cup soy milk
1/2 cup soy yogurt, vanilla flavor
1/4 tsp. cinnamon, ground

Method

1. Place the banana, silken tofu, soy milk, soy yogurt, and cinnamon in a blender. Process in until it becomes smooth.
2. Pour and divide among 2 chilled glasses. Sprinkle with more cinnamon on top, if desired.
3. Serve and enjoy!

Nutritional Information:

Energy – 160 kcal, Fat – 3.9 g, Carbs - 24.8 g, Protein – 8.1 g, Sodium – 52 mg

Strawberry Kiwi Milkshake

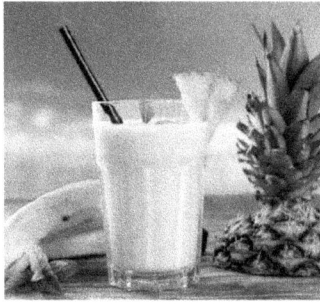

Preparation Time: 5 minutes**Yield:** 2 servings

Ingredients

1 cup pineapple, cubed
1 medium banana, sliced
6 oz. low-fat yogurt (vanilla flavor)
4-6 ice cubes
fresh mint sprigs

Method

1. Combine the pineapple, banana, yogurt, and ice cubes in a high-speed blender. Process until it becomes smooth.
2. Pour smoothie in 2 chilled glasses. Garnish with a small slice of pineapple and mint sprigs, if desired.
3. Serve immediately and enjoy.

Nutritional Information:

Energy – 154 kcal, Fat – 1.3 g, Carbs - 30.3 g, Protein – 5.9 g, Sodium – 61 mg

Berry Apple And Orange Smoothie

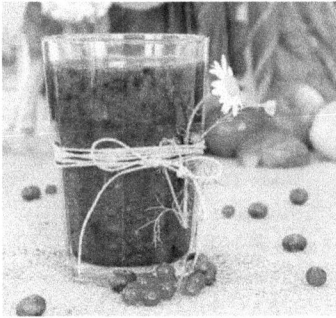

Preparation Time: 5 minutes**Yield:** 2 servings

Ingredients

1/2 cup blueberries
1/2 cup red currants
1 medium apple, cored and diced
1 medium seedless orange, peeled and cut into segments
6 oz. Greek yogurt
6 ice cubes

Method
1. Place the blueberries, red currants, apple, orange, yogurt, and ice cubes in a high-speed blender. Process until smooth.
2. Pour smoothie in 2 chilled glasses. Top with few berries, is desired.
3. Serve immediately and enjoy.

Nutritional Information:
Energy – 186 kcal, Fat – 1.5 g, Carbs - 35.0 g, Protein – 6.4 g, Sodium – 61 mg

Delicious And Healthy Green Smoothie

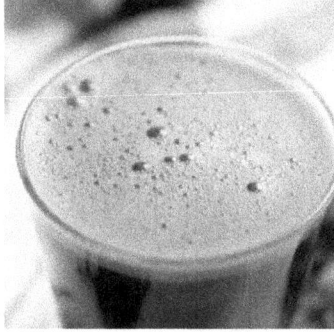

Preparation Time: 5 minutes**Yield:** 2 servings

Ingredients

1 medium apple, cored and diced
1 cup of chopped kale
1 cup of fresh orange juice
2 Tbsp. lemon juice
1 Tbsp. of flaxseeds
2 tsp. honey
1 cup ice cubes

Method
1. Place the apple, kale, orange juice, lemon juice, flaxseeds, honey, and ice cubes in a high-speed blender. Process until smooth.
2. Pour smoothie in 2 chilled glasses.

3. Serve immediately and enjoy.

Nutritional Information:
Energy – 156 kcal, Fat – 1.5 g, Carbs - 34.5 g, Protein – 3.1 g, Sodium – 20 mg

Black Currant Banana And Almond Smoothie

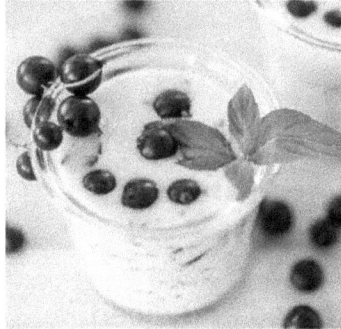

Preparation Time: 5 minutes**Yield:** 2 servings

Ingredients

1 cup black currants
2   medium   frozen   banana,   sliced
1 cup almond milk
1/4 tsp. pure vanilla extract
fresh mint sprigs

Method

1. Combine the black currants, banana, almond milk, and vanilla extract in a blender. Process until it becomes smooth.
2. Pour and divide smoothie among 2 chilled glasses. Garnish with few currants and mint sprigs.
3. Serve immediately and enjoy.

Nutritional Information:

Energy – 157 kcal, Fat – 1.9 g, Carbs - 32.1 g, Protein – 2.6 g, Sodium – 77 mg

Cardamom Raspberry And Pear Smoothie

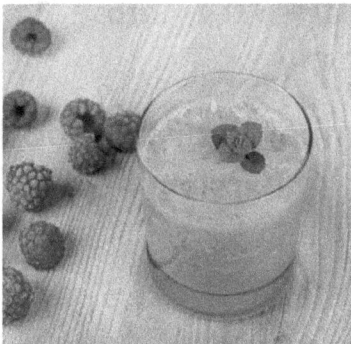

Preparation Time: 5 minutes**Yield:** 2 servings

Ingredients

1 cup fresh raspberries
1 medium pear, cored and diced
1 cup whole milk
1/4 tsp. cardamom
4 ice cubes
fresh mint sprigs

Method
1. Combine the raspberries, pear, milk, cardamom, and ice cubes in a blender. Process until it becomes smooth.
2. Pour smoothie in 2 chilled glasses. Garnish with mint sprigs.
3. Serve and enjoy.

Nutritional Information:
Energy – 134 kcal, Fat – 3.0 g, Carbs - 24.1 g, Protein – 5.0 g, Sodium – 59 mg

Banana Cucumber Radish Smoothie With Parsley

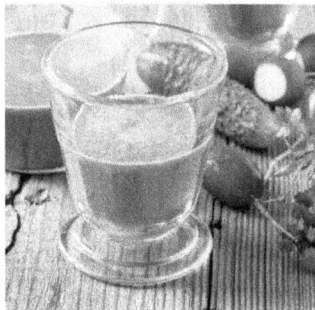

Preparation Time: 5 minutes**Yield:** 2 servings

Ingredients

1 medium frozen banana, sliced
1/2 medium cucumber, sliced
2 medium radishes, sliced
6 oz. Greek yogurt (plain)
1/2 cup organic rice milk

Method

1. Place the banana, cucumber, radish, yogurt, and rice milk in a high-speed blender. Process until smooth.
2. Pour smoothie in 2 chilled glasses.
3. Serve immediately and enjoy.

Nutritional Information:

Energy – 155 kcal, Fat – 1.8 g, Carbs - 28.6 g, Protein – 6.1 g, Sodium – 85 mg

Peach Banana And Cottage Cheese Smoothie

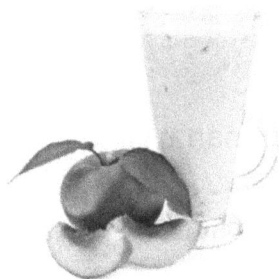

Preparation Time: 5 minutes**Yield:** 2 servings

Ingredients

2 peach halves, cut into small pieces
1 medium frozen banana, sliced
1 cup skim milk
1/2 cup cottage cheese
4 ice cubes

Method
1. Place the peach halves, banana, milk, cottage cheese, and ice cubes in a high-speed blender. Process until smooth and creamy.
2. Pour in 2 chilled glasses. Garnish with peach slices if desired.
3. Serve and enjoy.

Nutritional Information:

Energy – 178 kcal, Fat – 1.5 g, Carbs - 28.5 g, Protein – 13.1 g, Sodium – 195 mg

Kiwi Banana Smoothie With Pumpkin Seed

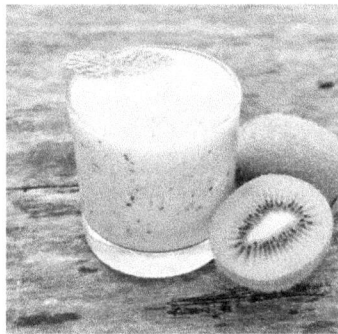

Preparation Time: 5 minutes**Yield:** 2 servings

Ingredients

1 cup kiwi fruit, peeled and cubed
1 medium banana, sliced
1 cup almond milk, unsweetened
1 cup ice cubes
2 Tbsp. pumpkin seeds
fresh mint sprigs

Method

1. Combine the kiwi, banana, almond milk, ice cubes, and pumpkin seeds in a high-speed blender. Process until it becomes smooth.
2. Pour smoothie in 2 chilled glasses. Garnish with mint sprigs.
3. Serve and enjoy.

Nutritional Information:

Energy – 168 kcal, Fat – 5.9 g, Carbs - 28.5 g, Protein – 4.3 g, Sodium – 80 mg

Raspberry Cucumber And Rhubarb Smoothie

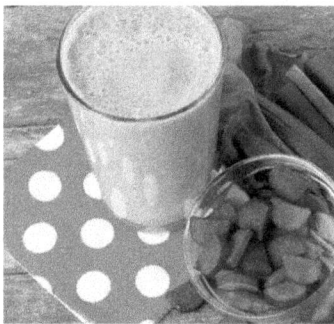

Preparation Time: 5 minutes **Yield:** 2 servings

Ingredients

1 cup frozen raspberries

1/2 medium cucumber (peeled, deseeded and cut into small pieces)
2 rhubarb (cut into small pieces)
1 cup almond milk, unsweetened
1 Tbsp. honey

Method

1. Combine the raspberries, cucumber, rhubarb, almond milk, and honey in a blender. Process until it becomes smooth.
2. Pour and divide smoothie among 2 chilled glasses.
3. Serve and enjoy!

Nutritional Information:

Energy – 103 kcal, Fat – 1.7 g, Carbs - 22.2 g, Protein – 2.3 g, Sodium – 78 mg

Purple Berry Smoothie

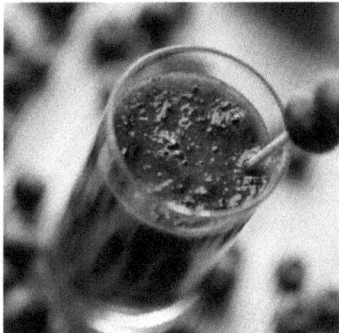

Preparation Time: 5 minutes**Yield:** 3 servings

Ingredients

2 cups blueberries
1 cup blackberries
1 cup cranberry juice
1 cup ice cubes

Method
1. Place the berries, cranberry juice, and ice cubes in a high-speed blender. Process until smooth.
2. Pour smoothie in 3 chilled glasses.
3. Serve and enjoy.

Nutritional Information:

Energy – 102 kcal, Fat – 0.6 g, Carbs - 22.4 g, Protein – 1.6 g, Sodium – 1 mg

Quick And Easy Fruit Cooler

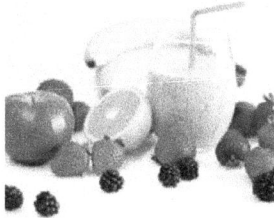

Preparation Time: 5 minutes**Yield:** 2 servings

Ingredients

1 medium apple, cored and diced
1/2 medium banana, sliced
1/2 cup strawberries
1/2 cup blackberries
1 cup whole milk
4-6 ice cubes

Method
1. Combine the apple, banana, strawberries, blackberries, milk, and ice cubes in a blender. Process until it becomes smooth.
2. Pour smoothie in chilled glasses.
3. Serve and enjoy.

Nutritional Information:

Energy – 154 kcal, Fat – 2.9 g, Carbs - 30.0 g, Protein –
5.6 g, Sodium – 59 mg

Fruit Cereal And Almond Smoothie

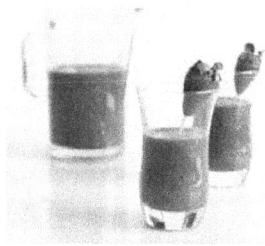

Preparation Time: 5 minutes**Yield:** 2 servings

Ingredients

1 cup almond milk
1 medium frozen banana, sliced
1/2 cup frozen strawberries
1/2 cup mango, diced
2 Tbsp. oat bran
2 Tbsp. wheat germ

Method
1. Combine the almond milk, banana, strawberries, mango, oat bran, and wheat germ in a blender. Process until smooth and creamy.
2. Pour smoothie in 2 chilled glasses. Garnish with strawberries, if desired.
3. Serve and enjoy.

Nutritional Information:

Energy – 149 kcal, Fat – 3.0 g, Carbs - 31.4 g, Protein – 5.1 g, Sodium – 77 mg

Luscious Banana-Mango Yogurt Smoothie

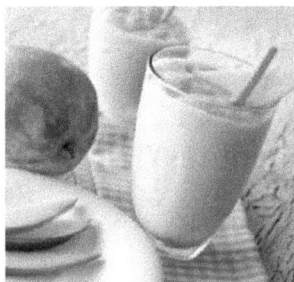

Preparation Time: 5 minutes**Yield:** 3 servings

Ingredients

1 medium banana, sliced
1 cup mango, diced
1 cup Greek yogurt
1 cup whole milk
1 cup ice cubes

Method

1. Place the banana, mango, yogurt, milk, and ice cubes in a high-speed blender. Process until smooth and creamy.

2. Pour and divide smoothie among 3 chilled glasses. Garnish with a small slice of mango and serve with straw, if desired.
3. Enjoy.

Nutritional Information:

Energy – 167 kcal, Fat – 3.0 g, Carbs - 27.1 g, Protein – 8.2 g, Sodium – 96 mg

Mango And Dragonfruit Smoothie

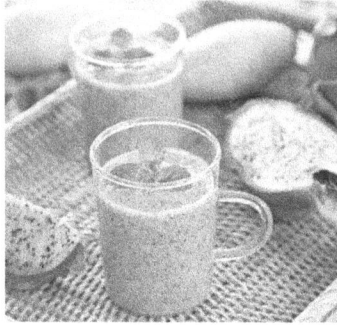

Preparation Time: 5 minutes**Yield:** 3 servings

Ingredients

2 medium dragonfruit
1 cup of mango, cubed
1 1/2 cup whole milk
1 Tbsp. chia seeds
1 cup ice cubes
fresh mint sprigs

Method
1. Combine the dragon fruit, mango, whole milk, chia seeds, and ice cubes in a blender. Process until it becomes smooth.
2. Pour smoothie in 3 chilled glasses. Garnish with fresh mint sprigs.
3. Serve immediately and enjoy.

Nutritional Information:

Energy – 157 kcal, Fat – 5.2 g, Carbs - 22.2 g, Protein – 6.6 g, Sodium – 99 mg

Pineapple Mango And Coconut Smoothie

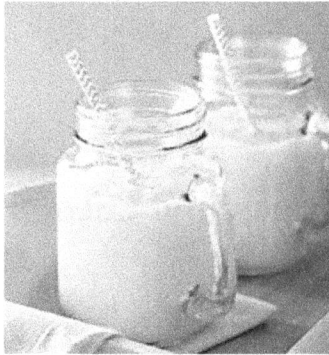

Preparation Time: 5 minutes**Yield:** 2 servings

Ingredients

1 cup pineapple, cubed
1 cup mango, diced
1 cup coconut water
1 cup ice cubes

Method

1. Combine the pineapple, mango, coconut water, and ice cubes in a blender. Process until it becomes smooth.
2. Pour the smoothie in 2 chilled glasses and serve with decorative straw, if desired.
3. Serve and enjoy.

Nutritional Information:

Energy – 113 kcal, Fat – 0.7 g, Carbs - 27.6 g, Protein – 2.0 g, Sodium – 128 mg

Pineapple Peach And Coconut Smoothie

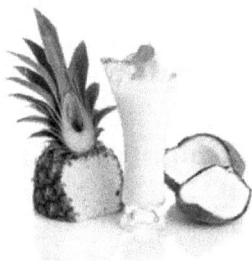

Preparation Time: 5 minutes**Yield:** 3 servings

Ingredients

1 cup frozen pineapple, cubed
1 medium frozen banana, sliced

2 peach halves, cubed
1 cup coconut water
1 cup ice cubes
1/3 cup coconut milk
1 Tbsp. honey

Method
1. Place the pineapple, banana, peach halves, coconut water, coconut milk, and honey in a blender. Process until smooth.
2. Pour smoothie in 3 chilled glasses and garnish with small slices of pineapple and peach, if desired.
3. Serve immediately and enjoy.

Nutritional Information:
Energy – 180 kcal, Fat – 6.9 g, Carbs - 31.1 g, Protein – 2.4 g, Sodium – 89 mg

Beet Dragon Fruit And Coconut Smoothie With Chia

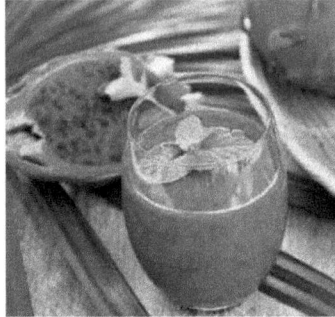

Preparation Time: 5 minutes**Yield:** 2 servings

Ingredients

2 medium beets, cut into small pieces
1 1/2 medium dragon fruit, peeled and diced
1 cup coconut water
1 cup crushed ice
1 Tbsp. chia seeds
fresh mint sprigs

Method
1. Combine the dragon fruit, beets, coconut water, ice, and chia in a blender. Process until it becomes smooth.
2. Pour smoothie in 2 chilled glasses. Garnish with fresh mint sprigs.

3. Serve and enjoy.

Nutritional Information:
Energy – 138 kcal, Fat – 3.7 g, Carbs - 22.1 g, Protein – 4.9 g, Sodium – 236 mg

Vegan Strawberry Smoothie With Walnuts

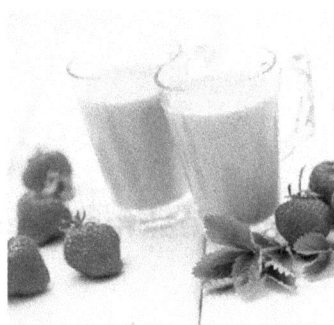

Preparation Time: 5 minutes**Yield:** 2 servings

Ingredients

1 ½ cups frozen strawberries
1 cup organic rice milk
1 tsp. maple syrup
1/4 cup chopped walnuts
fresh mint sprigs

Method

1. Place the strawberries, rice milk, maple syrup, and walnuts in a high-speed blender. Process until smooth.
2. Pour smoothie in 2 chilled glasses.
3. Serve immediately and enjoy.

Nutritional Information:

Energy – 193 kcal, Fat – 10.4 g, Carbs - 22.9 g, Protein – 4.5 g, Sodium – 44 mg

Cranberry Soy Breakfast Smoothie

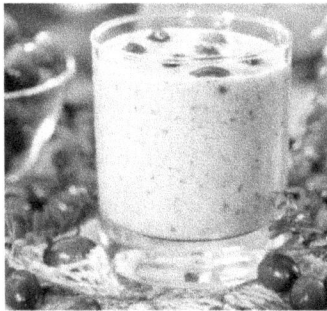

Preparation Time: 5 minutes**Yield:** 2 servings

Ingredients

1 cup frozen cranberries
6 oz. soy yogurt
1/2 cup soy milk
2 Tbsp. oat bran
1 Tbsp. wheat germ

Method
1. Place the cranberries, soy yogurt, soy milk, oat bran, and wheat germ in a blender. Process until it becomes smooth.
2. Pour smoothie in 2 chilled glasses. Garnish with few cranberries, if desired.
3. Serve immediately and enjoy.

Nutritional Information:
Energy – 161 kcal, Fat – 4.1 g, Carbs - 23.1 g, Protein – 7.7 g, Sodium – 39 mg

Dark Choco Banana And Peanut Butter Smoothie

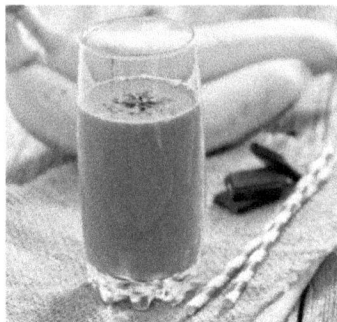

Preparation Time: 5 minutes**Yield:** 2 servings

Ingredients

1 1/2 cup almond milk, unsweetened
2 oz. melted dark chocolate
1 medium banana, sliced
1 Tbsp. peanut butter
1/2 cup crushed ice
chocolate shavings

Method
1. Place the almond milk, dark chocolate sauce, peanut butter, and crushed ice in a high-speed blender. Process until smooth.

2. Pour smoothie in 2 chilled glasses. Top with some chocolate shavings.
3. Serve immediately and enjoy.

Nutritional Information:

Energy – 230 kcal, Fat – 11.5 g, Carbs - 26.1 g, Protein – 4.5 g, Sodium – 182 mg

Watermelon Coconut Smoothie With Hemp Seed

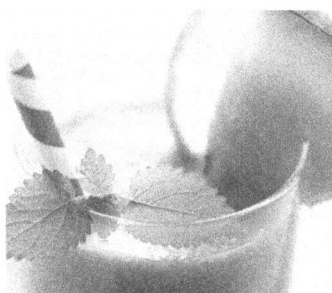

Preparation Time: 5 minutes**Yield:** 2 servings

Ingredients

1 ½ cups watermelon, cubed
1 cup coconut water
2 Tbsp. lemon juice
2 tsp. hemp seeds

2 tsp. agave nectar
4 ice cubes

Method

1. Combine the watermelon, coconut water, lemon juice, hemp seeds, agave nectar, and ice cubes in a blender. Process until mixture becomes smooth.
2. Pour smoothie in 2 chilled glasses.
3. Serve immediately and enjoy.

Nutritional Information:

Energy – 112 kcal, Fat – 2.2 g, Carbs - 21.6 g, Protein – 2.9 g, Sodium – 131 mg

Papaya Citrus Cooler With Honey

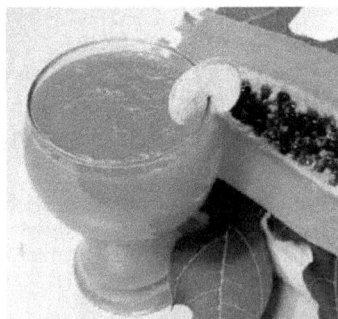

Preparation Time: 5 minutesYield: 2 servings

Ingredients

1 cup papaya, cubed
1 cup fresh orange juice
2 Tbsp. lime juice
1 Tbsp. honey
1 cup ice cubes

Method
1. Combine the papaya, orange juice, lime juice, honey, and ice cubes in a blender. Process until mixture becomes smooth.
2. Pour smoothie in 2 chilled glasses. Garnish with lime slices.
3. Serve and enjoy.

Nutritional Information:
Energy – 181 kcal, Fat – 3.6 g, Carbs – 29.4 g, Protein – 13.2 g, Sodium – 62 mg

Peach Strawberry And Almond Smoothie With Flax

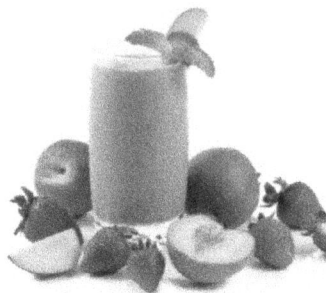

Preparation Time: 5 minutes**Yield:** 2 servings

Ingredients

2 peach halves, diced
1 cup fresh strawberries, halved
1 cup almond milk
1 Tbsp. flaxseeds
4-6 ice cubes

Method
1. Place the peach halves, strawberries, almond milk, flaxseeds, and ice cubes in a high-speed blender. Process until smooth and creamy.
2. Pour smoothie in 2 chilled glasses. Garnish with peach and strawberry slices, if desired.
3. Serve immediately and enjoy.

Nutritional Information:

Energy – 150 kcal, Fat – 3.1 g, Carbs - 28.1 g, Protein – 5.5 g, Sodium – 71 mg

Breakfast Choco Banana Protein Smoothie

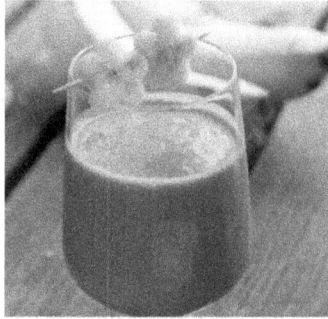

Preparation Time: 5 minutes**Yield:** 2 servings

Ingredients

2 scoops chocolate protein powder
1 medium frozen banana
2 cups almond milk
2 Tbsp. oat bran
1/4 tsp. cinnamon, ground

Method

1. Combine the chocolate powder, banana, almond milk, oat bran, and cinnamon in a blender and process until well blended and smooth.
2. Pour smoothie in 2 chilled glasses.
3. Serve immediately and enjoy.

Nutritional Information:

Energy – 151 kcal, Fat – 3.8 g, Carbs - 20.0 g, Protein – 12.5 g, Sodium – 231 mg

Avocado Soy And Maple Smoothie

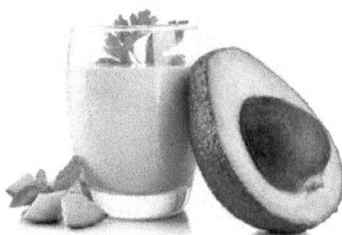

Preparation Time: 5 minutes**Yield:** 2 servings

Ingredients

1/2 cup avocado, diced
1 cup soy milk
1 cup crushed ice
1 Tbsp. maple syrup
fresh mint sprig

Method

1. Place the avocado, soy milk, crushed ice, and maple syrup in a high-speed blender. Process until smooth and creamy.
2. Pour smoothie in 2 chilled glasses. Garnish with mint sprig, if desired.
3. Serve immediately and enjoy.

Nutritional Information:

Energy – 167 kcal, Fat – 9.3 g, Carbs - 17.5 g, Protein – 4.7 g, Sodium – 66 mg

Strawberry Plum And Coconut Smoothie With Chia

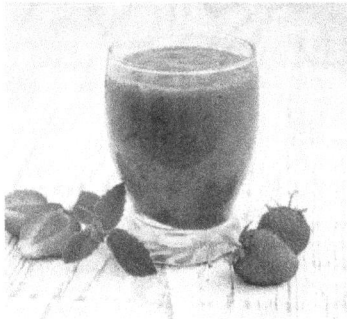

Preparation Time: 5 minutes**Yield:** 2 servings

Ingredients

1 cup strawberries
2 medium plum, pitted
1 1/2 cups coconut water
2 tsp. chia seeds
4-6 ice cubes

Method
1. Place the strawberries, plum, coconut water, chia seeds, and ice cubes in a blender. Process until it becomes smooth.
2. Pour smoothie in 2 chilled glasses.
3. Serve immediately and enjoy.

Nutritional Information:

Energy – 122 kcal, Fat – 3.0 g, Carbs - 23.2 g, Protein – 3.5 g, Sodium – 191 mg

Almond Choco Berry Smoothie

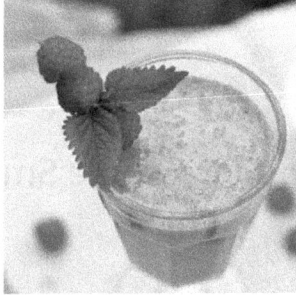

Preparation Time: 5 minutes**Yield:** 2 servings

Ingredients

2 cups frozen raspberries
2 Tbsp. chocolate syrup
1 cup almond milk, unsweetened
4 ice cubes

Method
1. Place raspberries, chocolate syrup, almond milk, and ice cubes in a blender. Process until mixture becomes smooth.
2. Pour in chilled glasses.
3. Serve and enjoy!

Nutritional Information:

Energy – 131 kcal, Fat – 2.3 g, Carbs - 27.4 g, Protein – 2.4 g, Sodium – 90 mg

Black Currant And Pineapple Smoothie With Chia

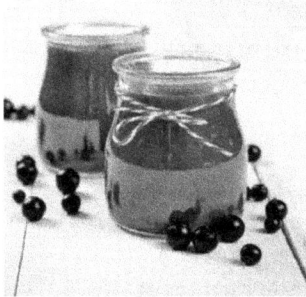

Preparation Time: 5 minutes**Yield:** 2 servings

Ingredients

1 cup black currants
1 cup pineapple, cubed
1/2 cup low-fat yogurt
1/2 cup skim milk
1 Tbsp. chia seeds

Method

1. Place black currants, pineapple, yogurt, milk, and chia seeds in a blender. Process until mixture becomes smooth.
2. Pour in chilled glasses.
3. Serve and enjoy!

Nutritional Information:

Energy – 177 kcal, Fat – 3.3 g, Carbs - 29.7 g, Protein – 7.9 g, Sodium – 79 mg

Raspberry Banana And Almond Smoothie

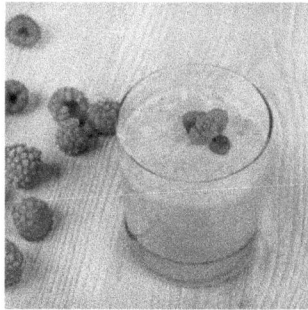

Preparation Time: 5 minutes**Yield:** 2 servings

Ingredients

1 1/2 cups raspberries
1 medium banana, sliced
1 1/2 cups almond milk

4 ice cubes

Method

1. Place raspberries, banana, almond milk, and ice cubes in a blender. Process until mixture becomes smooth.
2. Pour in chilled glasses.
3. Serve and enjoy!

Nutritional Information:

Energy – 123 kcal, Fat – 2.7 g, Carbs - 25.2 g, Protein – 2.5 g, Sodium – 114 mg

Banana Pear And Oat Smoothie

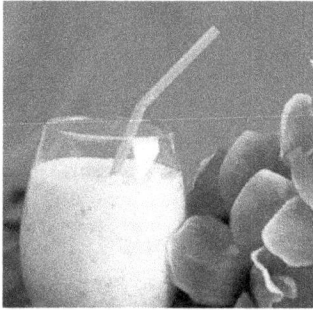

Preparation Time: 5 minutes**Yield:** 2 servings

Ingredients

1 medium banana, sliced
1 medium pear, cored and diced
2 Tbsp. rolled oats
1 cup whole milk
4 ice cubes

Method
1. Place banana, pear, rolled oats, milk, and ice cubes in a blender. Process until mixture becomes smooth.
2. Pour in chilled glasses.
3. Serve and enjoy!

Nutritional Information:

Energy – 185 kcal, Fat – 4.6 g, Carbs - 33.0 g, Protein – 5.5 g, Sodium – 51 mg

Berry Fruity Smoothie

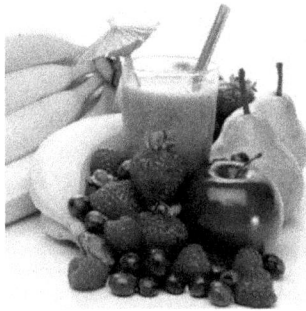

Preparation Time: 5 minutes**Yield:** 2 servings

Ingredients

1 cup frozen mixed berries
1/2 medium banana
1/2 medium apple
1/2 medium pear
1 cup skim milk

Method

1. Place mixed berries, banana, apple, pear, and skim milk in a blender. Process until mixture becomes smooth.
2. Pour in chilled glasses.
3. Serve and enjoy!

Nutritional Information:

Energy – 162 kcal, Fat – 0.5 g, Carbs - 36.2 g, Protein – 5.2 g, Sodium – 67 mg

Kiwi Banana And Mango Smoothie

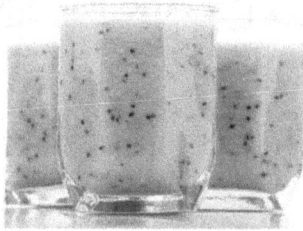

Preparation Time: 5 minutes**Yield:** 2 servings

Ingredients

1 medium kiwifruit
1/2 medium banana
1/2 cup mango

1 cup skim milk
4 ice cubes

Method
1. Place kiwifruit, banana, mango, milk, and ice cubes in a blender. Process until mixture becomes smooth.
2. Pour in chilled glasses.
3. Serve and enjoy!

Nutritional Information:

Energy – 137 kcal, Fat – 3.0 g, Carbs - 24.9 g, Protein – 5.2 g, Sodium – 58 mg

Berry Pineapple And Mango Smoothie

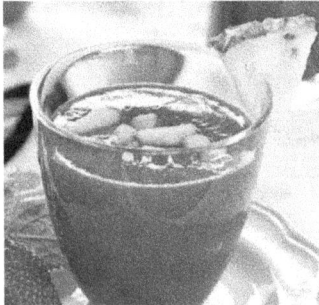

Preparation Time: 5 minutes**Yield:** 2 servings

Ingredients

1 cup strawberries
1 cup pineapple, cubed
1/2 cup mango, diced
1 cup almond milk, unsweetened
4 ice cubes

Method
1. Place strawberries, pineapple, mango, almond milk, and ice cubes in a blender. Process until mixture becomes smooth.
2. Pour in chilled glasses.
3. Serve and enjoy!

Nutritional Information:
Energy – 104 kcal, Fat – 1.7 g, Carbs - 23.0 g, Protein – 1.8 g, Sodium – 77 mg

Dragonfruit Mango And Almond Smoothie With Flax

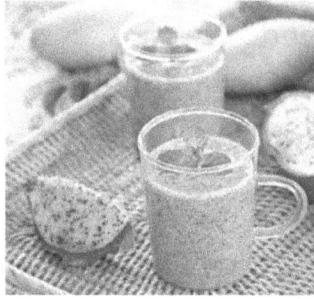

Preparation Time: 5 minutes**Yield:** 2 servings

Ingredients

1 medium dragonfruit
1 cup mango
1 1/2 cups almond milk, unsweetened
4 ice cubes

Method
1. Place dragonfruit, mango, almond milk, and ice cubes in a blender. Process until mixture becomes smooth.
2. Pour in chilled glasses.
3. Serve and enjoy!

Nutritional Information:

Energy – 102 kcal, Fat – 2.9 g, Carbs - 17.6 g, Protein – 2.4 g, Sodium – 143 mg

Dragonfruit Banana And Strawberry Smoothie

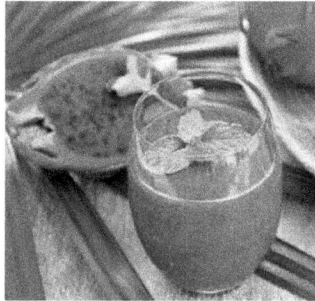

Preparation Time: 5 minutes**Yield:** 2 servings

Ingredients

1 medium dragonfruit
1 medium banana
1/2 cup strawberries
1 cup skim milk
4 ice cubes

Method

1. Place dragonfruit, banana, strawberries, milk, and ice cubes in a blender. Process until mixture becomes smooth.
2. Pour in chilled glasses.
3. Serve and enjoy!

Nutritional Information:

Energy – 139 kcal, Fat – 1.1 g, Carbs - 26.8 g, Protein – 5.9 g, Sodium – 96 mg

Strawberry Cheesecake Smoothie

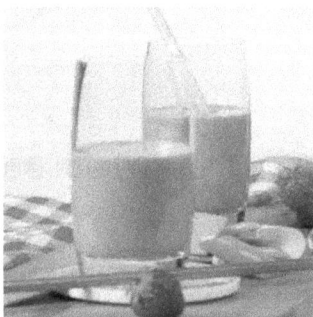

Preparation Time: 5 minutes**Yield:** 2 servings

Ingredients

2 cups strawberries
1/2 cup cottage cheese
1 cup skim milk
4 ice cubes

Method

1. Place strawberries, cottage cheese, milk, and ice cubes in a blender. Process until mixture becomes smooth.

2. Pour in chilled glasses.

3. Serve and enjoy!

Nutritional Information:

Energy – 142 kcal, Fat – 1.5 g, Carbs - 19.1 g, Protein – 12.7 g, Sodium – 291 mg

Orange Mango And Soy Smoothie

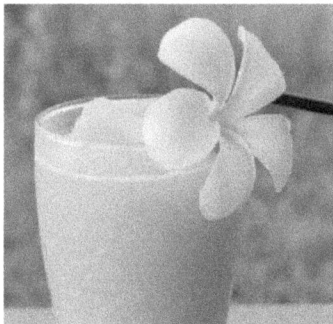

Preparation Time: 5 minutes**Yield:** 2 servings

Ingredients

1 medium orange
1 cup mango
1 cup soy milk, unsweetened
4 ice cubes

Method
1. Place kiwifruit, banana, mango, milk, and ice cubes in a blender. Process until mixture becomes smooth.
2. Pour in chilled glasses.
3. Serve and enjoy!

Nutritional Information:
Energy – 146 kcal, Fat – 2.5 g, Carbs - 27.8 g, Protein – 5.3 g, Sodium – 63 mg

Blackberry Cheesecake Smoothie

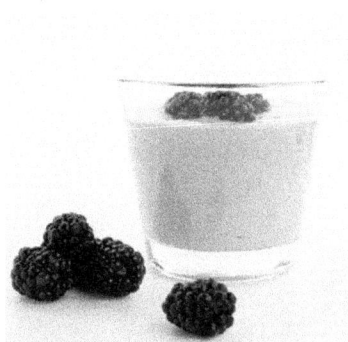

Preparation Time: 5 minutes**Yield:** 2 servings

Ingredients

2 cups blackberries
1/2 cup cottage cheese
1 cup skim milk
4 ice cubes

Method
1. Place blackberries, cottage cheese, milk, and ice cubes in a blender. Process until mixture becomes smooth.
2. Pour in chilled glasses.
3. Serve and enjoy!

Nutritional Information:

Energy – 158 kcal, Fat – 1.8 g, Carbs - 21.9 g, Protein – 13.8 g, Sodium – 296 mg

Raspberry Soy Yogurt Smoothie With Hemp

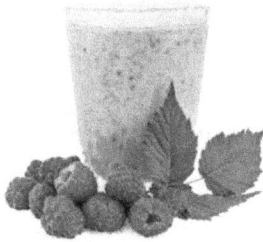

Preparation Time: 5 minutes**Yield:** 2 servings

Ingredients

2 cups raspberries
1 cup soy milk, unsweetened
1 tsp. hemp seeds
4 ice cubes

Method

1. Place raspberries, soy milk, hemp seeds, and ice cubes in a blender. Process until mixture becomes smooth.
2. Pour in chilled glasses.
3. Serve and enjoy!

Nutritional Information:

Energy – 151 kcal, Fat – 4.7 g, Carbs - 22.6 g, Protein – 6.7 g, Sodium – 64 mg

Mango Passion Smoothie With Chia

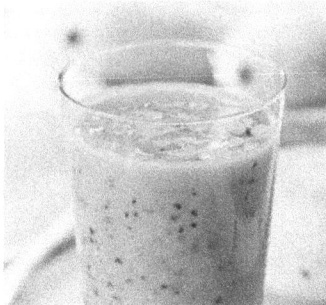

Preparation Time: 5 minutes**Yield:** 2 servings

Ingredients

1 cup mango
1/2 cup passion fruit
2 cups almond milk, unsweetened
1 Tbsp. chia seeds

Method
1. Place mango, passion fruit, almond milk, and chia seeds in a blender. Process until mixture becomes smooth.
2. Pour in chilled glasses.
3. Serve and enjoy!

Nutritional Information:
Energy – 171 kcal, Fat – 5.4 g, Carbs - 30.1 g, Protein – 4.2 g, Sodium – 168 mg

Coco Banana And Citrus Smoothie

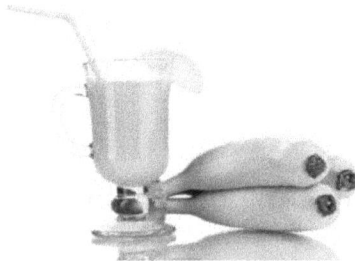

Preparation Time: 5 minutes**Yield:** 2 servings

Ingredients

1 medium frozen banana
1 medium orange
1/4 cup coconut milk
1 cup coconut water

Method
1. Place banana, orange, coconut milk, coconut water, and ice cubes in a blender. Process until mixture becomes smooth.
2. Pour in chilled glasses.
3. Serve and enjoy!

Nutritional Information:
Energy – 175 kcal, Fat – 7.7 g, Carbs - 27.3 g, Protein – 2.8 g, Sodium – 131 mg

Blueberry Banana And Coconut Smoothie

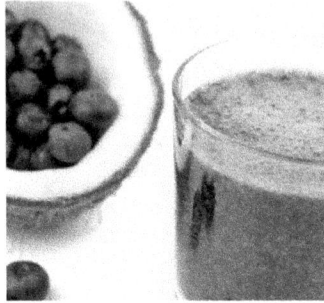

Preparation Time: 5 minutes**Yield:** 2 servings

Ingredients

1 cup frozen blueberries
1 medium frozen banana
1/4 cup coconut milk
1 cup coconut water

Method
1. Place blueberries, banana, coconut milk, and coconut water in a blender. Process until mixture becomes smooth.
2. Pour in chilled glasses.
3. Serve and enjoy!

Nutritional Information:

Energy – 186 kcal, Fat – 7.8 g, Carbs - 30.1 g, Protein – 2.7 g, Sodium – 132 mg

Strawberry Yogurt And Oat Smoothie

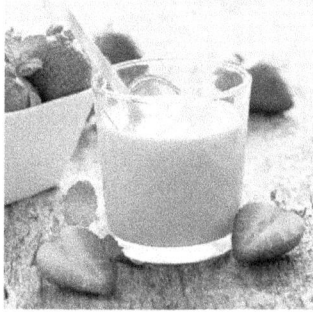

Preparation Time: 5 minutes**Yield:** 2 servings

Ingredients

1 cup frozen strawberries
1 cup vanilla or plain Greek yogurt
1/2 cup skim milk
2 Tbsp. rolled oats

Method

1. Place strawberries, yogurt, milk, and rolled oats in a blender. Process until mixture becomes smooth.
2. Pour in chilled glasses.
3. Serve and enjoy!

Nutritional Information:

Energy – 152 kcal, Fat – 2.1 g, Carbs - 20.6 g, Protein – 10.1 g, Sodium – 119 mg

Blueberry Pear And Almond Smoothie

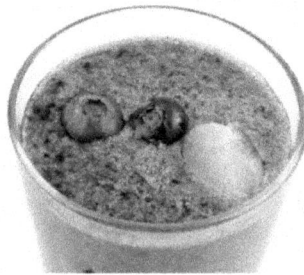

Preparation Time: 5 minutes**Yield:** 2 servings

Ingredients

1 cup frozen blueberries

1 medium pear
1 1/2 cups almond milk, unsweetened
1 Tbsp. honey
4 ice cubes

Method
1. Place blueberries, pear, almond milk, honey, and ice cubes in a blender. Process until mixture becomes smooth.
2. Pour in chilled glasses.
3. Serve and enjoy!

Nutritional Information:
Energy – 136 kcal, Fat – 2.2 g, Carbs - 30.5 g, Protein – 1.6 g, Sodium – 114 mg

Sweet Berry And Banana Smoothie

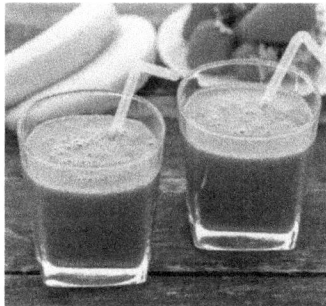

Preparation Time: 5 minutes**Yield:** 2 servings

Ingredients

1 cup frozen strawberries
1 medium frozen banana
1 1/2 cups skim milk
1 Tbsp. honey

Method
1. Place strawberries, banana, milk, and honey in a blender. Process until mixture becomes smooth.
2. Pour in chilled glasses.
3. Serve and enjoy!

Nutritional Information:
Energy – 175 kcal, Fat – 0.4 g, Carbs - 36.7 g, Protein – 7.2 g, Sodium – 99 mg